The War on Doctors

And the Destruction of US Healthcare

Linda Girgis, MD, FAAFP

Dedication

For those who struggle to give the patients their best, every day, even when no one is watching. There are still heroes among us.

Table of Contents

Preface

Walking the hospital corridors, many of the comments I overhear from patients and others speaking about doctors amaze me. One day, I took notice of the conversation between two elderly women who were none too happy with doctors, whom they stated only cared about their computers these days and not about their patients.

Upon hearing this, I wanted to scream out that nothing is further from the reality of what doctors truly feel. In fact, many days, a burning desire to toss my computer out the second floor window consumes me, but I rein it in. Doctors abhor spending time during the patient visit on their computers, documenting in the electronic chart. This decision was foisted on us, much against our wills, by governmental mandates. EHR (or electronic health record) technology was forced upon us, as well as its antecedent, meaningful use requirements. If we do not comply, we will be financially penalized, so we have little choice. I have published many articles on this topic.

Patients do not see this, however. They want our time; they need our eye contact; they need to know we care about their health. They do not want us keyboarding away while they open their hearts to us. It makes them feel insecure. It lets mistrust sneak in. This lack of trust is very harmful to the doctor-patient relationship in many ways. Perhaps the most important is that patients are less likely to follow our medical advice when the trust is not there. This can lead to unfavorable medical outcomes.

Reading or watching the media now exemplifies the anti-doctor culture now prevalent in the US. Even in a State of the Union Address, our own President Barack Obama suggested that doctors perform procedures for profit. He completely disregarded the integrity of most doctors who work long hours, studied for many years, and make every effort to give patients our very best care. The media clamors for us to be transparent about our charges, while many of us close our doors because we can no longer afford to practice. We see the stereotype the media portrays of us: greedy doctors driven by profit. Yet, how many of those journalists volunteered to visit our practices or even talk to us and see what it is like in the exam room and what we deal with on a daily basis? It is far easier just to perpetuate a stereotype than to investigate the reality. Sure, there exist some greedy doctors out there. However, the truth is, the majority of doctors despise them because they give us all a bad name and cast us in an unfavorable light. Does anyone want to know what the average doctor is like? Or do we just want to hate them all in the same way because it pleases us?

The war on doctors flames in boardrooms across the country, as healthcare executives discuss how to profit off our work. They place no value on our expertise, but rather calculate how they can reduce our reimbursements and get us to practice medicine in the way they desire to reduce costs and maximize their revenue. Doctors are not judged by clinical skills but rather by how much money they saved for the insurance company. I receive these analyses quarterly from many of the insurance companies that I contract with. If I prevent my patients from going to the Emergency Department (ED) to obtain medical care or only prescribe them the cheapest medications, I earn a higher rating. Do we want to be treated by doctors who know how to cut costs the most, or by those with the best medical skills and knowledge? Sure, we all need to be conscious of healthcare costs, but not by sacrificing the best care for our patients. Insurance companies see their bottom lines. I, and most physicians, see a patient in front of us in the exam room that we want to help, to cure, to heal, and to prevent a bad outcome from happening. All too often, the insurance company often overrides our medical decisions in order to save costs, not lives. How has the system lost its priority like this?

The government is no ally to doctors either. All too frequently in recent years, laws and mandates have been pouring forth from the halls of the House and Senate, putting more restrictions on doctors. These mandates do little to improve patient outcomes. There is no evidence available that they do, yet doctors are forced to comply with these regulations or face

The War on Doctors

financial penalties. In fact, if you look further into these new laws—for example, MU, PQRS, PCMH—it appears that these systems are just a way for the government to have an easy way to harvest more data about our patients. Do we really want that? Why is the government turning patients into data? In the future, doctors will be paid if patients meet certain clinical outcomes, like target LDL cholesterol levels, BP readings, and many more. Shouldn't we be worried about the whole person and their health rather than aiming for a specific target number? The governmental mandates are changing all this. To make matters worse, the government is the one establishing these guidelines. Do we really want our politicians deciding what is best for our health more than doctors do? Isn't it time politicians removed themselves from practicing medicine unless they have earned a medical degree?

Unless we stand up and demand changes, we are facing a future where the doctor no longer has much input into your medical care. They will be forced to follow guidelines established by those without any formal medical training. Patients will be the biggest losers in this new medical world. They will no longer be a player in their own healthcare decisions. They will be relegated to what their insurance companies allow them to receive, based on cost alone. There will be no more private doctors or small practices. Patients will only be able to see doctors if they are lucky, in large systems, or hospital groups. They will no longer have a personal relationship with their doctor, who will now just be a cog in the wheel, signing off only on what he is allowed. The patient will become a number, like at the deli counter—patient in, patient out. The patient will leave dissatisfied because they had to pay for the visit because of their high deductible. They were not able to receive any medications or tests they needed because the insurance company denied them...and they were too expensive to pay out-of-pocket. The doctor will be burnt out and the patient disgruntled. The government will have the data they need because the burnt-out doctor is forced to submit it under financial penalty. The insurance company maximized their profits, with their CEOs and other administrators making annual salaries in the tens of millions of dollars (as already happens in the present day).

3

Linda Girgis

These are historic times for the US healthcare system. We are watching it destruct before our very eyes. The days of Marcus Welby-type medicine are long gone. Yes, these are historic times in medicine as the curtain closes on the way we have trained and learned to practice medicine. The doctor is no longer center stage, unless you are watching a puppet show. We are now the supporting cast. Patients no longer have center stage, either. The stars are the CEOs, the administrators who are raking in the big bucks and determining company guidelines and what doctors can and cannot do. The co-stars are the politicians, who issue mandates for their own gain, to push their own agendas and to line their own pockets.

The war on doctors is flaming. The American healthcare system is being destroyed.
Are we going to fight back? Or are we going to watch history unfold?

First published on drlinda-md.com

The War on Doctors

Chapter 1 The Media War on Doctors

When anyone watches or reads the news, there are stories of outrage pouring forth about mistaken surgeries or medication errors and how patients were harmed. These are very real concerns and need to be addressed. However, they are not as common as the media leads us to believe. Rarely do we witness tales of lives saved or the doctors who stay awake nights on end caring for others. No one seems interested to know how doctors sacrifice family time to provide patients medical care at all hours of the day. This media war is really an attack on the knowledge, skill set, and compassion of doctors.

Recent years revealed more stories of "pill mill" doctors. It seems the media is drawn to these types of stories. Apparently, there was one such doctor practicing not so far from me. The patient in front of me was asking if I read the newspaper and saw how this doctor was arrested. I knew the tale because I saw a whole string of new patients looking for prescriptions for controlled substances. They all became rather aggressive when I refused, as is my policy, to give it to them. The story of this doctor played out for weeks in local media, and patients believed that all doctors prescribed like he did. The flip side of the coin was not given coverage. They did not show how the majority of doctors fight this battle in their exam rooms every day. Most doctors walk out with their integrity intact and do not give in to the demands of obviously drug-seeking patients.

In a popular *Slate* article last year, it was discussed how doctors use the term SHPOS (subhuman piece of s^&^%) for difficult patients we don't like. In fact, the article states, "the term is known to physicians everywhere, passed by word of mouth from resident to intern to medical student."[1] Reading this article, the reader is given the impression that this is a common medical acronym used by doctors in derision to discuss patients we hate. I never heard this term before reading this *Slate* article. Perhaps I missed that part of my medical training? In fact, most doctors have never heard this acronym either. According to doctors polled on

SERMO (the largest social network exclusive to physicians), 91% reported that they had never heard this acronym. Additionally, 73% felt that this type of article harms the medical profession.

One can see how this negative article can paint doctors in a bad light and how it doesn't even need to pass a litmus test of accuracy. Anyone who read that article would be led to believe that all doctors use this offensive acronym to talk about patients. No, we do not. Any doctor who does should be reprimanded. It is never acceptable to refer to another human being, especially a patient who has trusted us with their health, in such a disgraceful manner. I teach many residents and medical students and they would never be allowed to speak thus in my presence. Sure, there are difficult patients and I doubt anyone would disagree with that. If there is a problem patient, call them what they are: difficult, angry, resentful, but please do not be so foul as to ever refer to a patient as a SHPOS. This is not acceptable and the vast majority of doctors agree. Too bad this reporter didn't research the truth before casting us in such a disgraceful light.

In another article in *The Atlantic,* published in November 2014 ("Doctors Tell All—And It's Bad"), the author relates her tale of suffering a chronic disease while going without a diagnosis for over a decade. According to her, physicians were "brusque and even hostile" and in the hospital, "the lighting was bad, the food terrible, the rooms loud." When she was finally diagnosed with Lyme disease, she states that she was right and the doctors were all wrong. While what she suffered is terrible, she did get relief in the healthcare system. Yet, she denounces the whole system, describing it as an "emotionally deficient and inconsistent medical system that is best at treating acute, not chronic problems." She further states that the system is full of "countless cases of substandard care, overlooked diagnoses, bureaucratic bungling, and even outright antagonism between doctor and patient." She told of ER workers barely registering human distress and that fee-for-service rewards doctors for doing as many services as possible rather than providing good care. It was alleged that stressed-out doctors directly take out their frustrations on their patients.[2] While Meghan O'Rourke does touch on some of the problems inherent in the US healthcare system, she paints a doom-and-

The War on Doctors

gloom picture with all doctors being substandard and un-empathetic. No one reading this would believe that there are good doctors in the system. I doubt there are any other articles in the mainstream media showing the opposite point-of-view. Yes, there are poor care and problems in the system. However, there are many good doctors and healthcare workers who sacrifice much to give their patients the very best. These types of articles are important to report, but without citing the positive that exists, we are seeing only an overly dramatized picture. In a decade of seeking treatment, I am sure the author saw some of the positives as well. But again, the media loves to demonize doctors.

It saddens me to see so many people believe that doctors are driven by greed and making money. Claims are made in the media that doctors do procedures just for profit, even by our Commander-in-Chief President Obama. I am sure most remember his statement that doctors make more money performing tonsillectomies than with conservative treatment. However, for the majority of doctors, nothing could be further from reality.

Doctors are battling many forces every day on behalf of our patients, many that will never be seen or be appreciated. There are the prior authorization and prescription refills that fill our days. We are always available after hours, whether personally or with a shared coverage group. All this work is uncompensated but we do it for the sake of our patients. We do it because this is what they need to have the best care.

Patients don't know how much we truly care about them. Sometimes we stay awake all night worrying that they will be all right until the morning. They don't see us on Christmas morning as we are watching our own children opening their gifts, which we cast aside to answer their call because their child is vomiting. This is our calling. This is what we are supposed to do, because we do care about this other child and want them to be well.

We sometimes can feel the fear that is in a patient's eyes, fear of what terrible disease may be lurking inside. We try to stand up to that fear and calm it down. Sometimes it breaks us down. Sometimes, medicine fails and there is nothing left to offer. Sometimes, doctors go and cry alone because we take the failure of the medical field as our own.

Each patient is unique to us. That is why we balk so much at following set guidelines. Each patient needs to be evaluated for who they are and not how they fit on a clinical pathway. It would be much easier to just follow these care plans, but we care and our patients deserve our best-personalized care.

We feel when our patients die, no matter how old and how sick. We are amazed at their fortitude despite suffering. We learn from their strong spirits. We know their passing is a loss to the world and a tragedy to their loved ones. There may be some outlier doctors who are driven by greed, but this is a tiny minority. Most doctors truly care. There are many services we do free, just because we do care, not because we expect any payment in return. When everyone goes to bed at night, there is always a doctor standing by if they are needed.

In another article in *The Daily Beast* in 2014, there was a discussion on "How Being a Doctor Became the Most Miserable Profession." This article states that "being a doctor has become a miserable and humiliating undertaking" and discloses that 9 out of 10 doctors would tell others not to join the profession. According to this article, people see certain specialists, such as ophthalmologists as "making out like bandits" and scorn such doctors. It additionally asserts that being a primary care doctor "is more like being a janitor".[3] Ouch! So much for my specialty. The remainder of this article discusses how doctors got to this state. Honestly, I love being a doctor and a primary care physician. Despite what the media says, being a physician is still a noble profession. There is no other career that gives us the opportunity to save lives and make a difference to such a great degree in the wellbeing of others. Many doctors I do know still love their profession as well.

A *USA Today* article from August 2013 tells us that thousands of doctors are practicing despite medical errors and misconduct. This article outlines the wrong action of one doctor specifically and does present statistics of

The War on Doctors

the wrongdoing of doctors. It states that these numbers came from several sources, yet fails to cite all of them. This article states, "Despite years of criticism, the nation's state medical boards continue to allow thousands of physicians to keep practicing medicine after findings of serious misconduct that put patients at risk." [4] It does not disclose where this information came from specifically or if these were closed or open cases. It does not state if these doctors were disciplined or if the allegations were determined to be unfounded. We are not given a true picture, only the sensationalism of the bad doctor harming patients that the media and public seem to love.

Yes again, there are doctors who do bad things. No one is arguing that point. However, just reading media accounts is misleading and gives us a bad impression of all doctors. These articles lack balance by failing to show that the good doctors do far outweigh these other incidences. Sure, they should be reported, but be fair and balanced and be accurate in the report.

An article in *Slate* describes for us how doctors are bullies and throw fits. Apparently, there is an epidemic of bullying doctors who harm nurses and put patients' lives in jeopardy. This article focuses on a book that reveals the stories of four nurses and interviews of "hundreds of other nurses." So, what is considered bullying? Of those polled, 87% reported that doctors had a "reluctance to answer your questions or return calls." I am not sure if many would agree that this constitutes bullying. Perhaps the doctor was just thinking of the proper response? Other stats show how many nurses were talked to in a condescending fashion or had objects thrown at them. Of course, these are unprofessional behaviors and should not be tolerated by anyone and other doctors should be the first to police these horrors. This article makes out that there is a grand organizational conspiracy to silence the fact that doctors are bullies. There is no conspiracy here. The article concludes that nurses are to be respected and should not put up with this behavior. [5] I absolutely agree. Doctors who fume and throw things should not be tolerated. However, the remaining doctors should be respected as well and not be made out to be bandits. Are there doctors who are bullies? Sure there are, but the majority are not.

I could keep going on with the media war on doctors and how we are being demonized. Stories abound of patients who went in to undergo wisdom tooth extraction and died or had the wrong surgery performed on them. We need to hear these stories. I think they can actually be helpful to patients to know that all procedures carry certain risks. Bariatric surgery, for example, is not the magic weight loss procedure that will make you lose weight safely. People suffer complications from it. Patients should hear real stories when making their medical decisions. Do medical errors happen in hospitals? Recent statistics are clearly telling us yes. These stories may make patients into stronger advocates for themselves, knowing these risks are out there.

However, the media accounts of doctors sensationalize these stories without giving balanced accounts. The media wants to diabolize us. It is not just doctors doing badly, but we all know bad news brings attention, like those who crane their necks at the sight of car accidents. I suppose it is just human nature. Doctors are struggling these days. We are fighting wars on many fronts. Perhaps the media battle is the most harmful in the sense that we are vilified and the public loses its trust in us. To be fair, patients can put any stories out in the public that they choose. Doctors, on the other hand, are prohibited from defending themselves against these allegations due to HIPAA laws. Patients' confidentiality needs to be respected at all costs, even when our reputations are being damaged. The silence of doctors does not imply their guilt. It may signify their dedication to protect patient privacy. As we fight this war on the public media front, does the public want the full truth, or just the means of flogging physicians? Isn't it time we rebuild the trust and come a team again?

1. http://www.slate.com/articles/health_and_science/medical_exa miner/2014/11/sub_human_pos_doctors_acronym_for_the_wor st_patients_is_shpos.html
2. http://www.theatlantic.com/magazine/archive/2014/11/doctors-tell-all-and-its-bad/380785/

The War on Doctors

3. http://www.thedailybeast.com/articles/2014/04/14/how-being-a-doctor-became-the-most-miserable-profession.html
4. http://www.usatoday.com/story/news/nation/2013/08/20/doctors-licenses-medical-boards/2655513/
5. http://www.slate.com/articles/health_and_science/medical_examiner/2015/04/doctors_bully_nurses_hospital_mistreatment_is_a_danger_to_patient_health.single.html

Chapter 2 Third-Party Power Plays

The patient was a 17-year-old boy, star of his high school basketball team. He was afflicted with asthma all his life that was made worse with exercise. He had done fairly well as long as he pre-medicated himself prior to exertion with his inhaler. Unfortunately for him, under the new health insurance exchange plans, many companies altered their formularies to no longer cover asthma inhalers, even generic ones. He ran out of his medication, had a severe exacerbation, and landed in the ER. Thankfully, he received appropriate treatment and a sample inhaler, although not the best medication for him, and was advised to follow up with me. Now, all would be well if we could just get him back on his usual inhaler that kept him symptom-free for years.

That is when the war began. This patient could not afford to pay $70 a month for a generic inhaler. His mother was raising him and his siblings alone and there was no extra money. She was scraping by to give them the best and he was struggling to keep up his grades and hopefully land a basketball scholarship. This family was doing what they were supposed to be doing, yet were unable to receive appropriate and even simple care. Instead of covering a $70 inhaler, they ended up covering a $1000+ ED visit. Does anyone see where the cost savings come in here?

Of course, this boy would be perfectly fine if he could just get the insurance company to pay for his inhaler that they had covered for years. We went to the next step of doing the dreaded prior-authorization. The insurance company staff on the phone fighting the battle has no medical training whatsoever. Her only goal is to deny that inhaler to cut costs and protect her job. My only goal is to get that medication so that my patient can be able to breathe. After much instruction from her about their formulary issues, I went into an education dissertation on the mechanism of airway obstruction and inflammation in asthma and why my patient might *die* without his inhaler and she would be responsible. She has no clue what I was saying; in fact, she asked me to spell several of the words and handed me off to a supervisor.

The War on Doctors

The next stage in the battle ensued until finally I landed a victorious peer-to-peer review with the medical director. Two hours after this battle ensued, the boy walked to his pharmacy to claim his authorized generic asthma inhaler so that he could continue to breathe. No one would know how much time I spent on the phone completing that task in between seeing a waiting room full of patients.

Increasingly, third parties control more of the practice of medicine. They decide the formularies of what medications a patient is allowed to have. They develop guidelines that decide what tests a patient is permitted to have done and when and where it is to be done. Doctors are losing the power to make medical decisions. The patients are no longer a part of the team but rather a pawn that the insurance companies use to drive profits. Insurance companies are not regulated. They are not required to cover medical treatments, no matter how much of a premium a person pays them. They can change their guidelines at any time without any oversight or liability.

So who is really making healthcare decisions and how does this play out? One example was a patient with severe shoulder pain. The patient in the exam room needed his wife and daughter to help him put his shirt back on. He was physically unable to do so by himself because he was unable to raise his shoulder high enough to do so.

My diagnostic impression led me to believe that he had a rotator cuff tear and would need surgery to repair it. From past clinical experiences, I knew I could get him in to see an orthopedist more quickly if I had a MRI confirming the diagnosis rather than referring him with shoulder pain.

In the past, this was indeed the way the medical course would progress and the patient would be in quickly for treatment to alleviate his suffering. But not this time, and not many times in recent months.

The medical treatment halted when the patient's medical insurance company deemed the MRI not medically necessary.

I think we all understand that insurance companies have staff hired to follow certain clinical pathways to control costs and maximize company profits. Many do not possess any medical training or even any advanced training other than a high school diploma. However, all that aside, I took the next step and appealed to medical reason, the medical director.

The insurance companies now call these peer-to-peer discussions because, in theory, we are equally educated. In the past, I have often reasoned with these medical directors to see the medical decision from my point of view.

However, there was no reasoning in this "peer-to-peer" discussion. According to company clinical guidelines, the patient had to try six weeks of physical therapy first and fail.

In my mind, that equals six weeks of torture for a patient who cannot raise his shoulder enough to dress himself, comb his hair, or brush his teeth with his dominant hand. My pleas fell on deaf ears and in the end, the medical director explained that she was not denying care and the patient was free to pay for the MRI out-of-pocket.

Of course, the patient was currently unable to work without the use of his shoulder so had no extra money to pay for such an expensive test. The quicker he received treatment, the sooner he would be back to work and off disability.

If we disregard compassion and true medical care and go with insurance company guidelines (i.e., cost containment), this does not make sense either. Over time, leaving this patient untreated will cost more in terms of disability, pain medications, doctors' visits, wife's time lost at work to take care for his needs and many more. Through faulty insurance company reasoning, the costs were driven up rather than being contained.

So, who made the medical decision here?

My medical decision was to have the patient do an MRI to confirm the diagnosis and then to go on and be treated as soon as possible by an orthopedist. My decision was based on the history I gathered from speaking with the patient and from my physical examination, as well as my past experience treating similar patients.

The decision here was made by the medical director based on insurance company guidelines to control costs, without ever speaking to the patient or examining him. Yet, I am the one responsible for that decision. The medical director is pretty much held free from liability by contractual terms. She is free to make these decisions every day with no oversight like doctors in the trenches must face.

I ask again, who is really making the medical decisions about our patients? Shouldn't they at least share the liability or at least bear the responsibility of their own actions like the rest of us do?

Increasingly, I am seeing coverage for medical tests being denied. Patients are becoming increasingly disenfranchised by their plans as they are paying more into the premiums and higher copays. All too often, insurance companies are asking for prior-authorizations for services to be rendered and all too often, they result in denials. I sometimes spend days in the battle of prior-authorizations trying to get a needed test ordered. Many times, I end up in a phone battle with the medical director of any given insurance company. Most often, they understand what my patients need and will give approval. In recent weeks, denials have been more common. These decisions are determined by someone who has had no direct contact with my patient or even spoken with them.

Of course, they always say that they are just determining medical coverage and not practicing medical care on my patient. They state that the patient is still free to get the test; they will just have to pay for it themselves. My patients cannot afford these costly tests, so yes, it is making a medical determination for them. That is why they have insurance coverage. If they could afford their own medical care, they wouldn't need insurance. Many Americans are depending on their coverage for their medical wellbeing. There is an agreement there that is being violated. Patients are not getting what they pay for.

This is not happening in regard to just diagnostic tests but also prescription coverage as well. In the past few weeks, I have had several patients with hypertension not be able to get their usual medications refilled because the formulary suddenly changed. They were unable to pay out-of-pocket because the cost was unaffordable even for generics, not a cheap medication by any means. As anyone knows, these medications are life-saving. No person should end up in the ER while these prior-authorization games are happening.

These prior-authorizations are indeed harmful. How?

1. They delay needed treatment. Someone may have a life-threatening disease that cannot wait 3 days while the insurance company renders a decision. This delay is frankly putting lives at risk.
2. The delay slows down the process of finding the correct diagnosis. Sometimes tests need to be done just to rule out certain diseases before other tests can be done. The prior-auths slow down the whole process, delaying correct diagnosis and prompt treatment. Rare disease patients are especially being adversely affected by this process. Often, their disease is so rare that no clinical guidelines exist.
3. Not knowing a diagnosis increases patients' anxiety and fear. Doesn't everyone want to know what is wrong with them as soon as possible? Many people lose nights of sleep worrying about this. Don't they deserve a timely diagnosis?
4. It erodes the doctor-patient relationship. Many patients just don't understand prior-auths and think the delay comes from the doctor. There is nothing further from the truth. Doctors spend hours in these battles when the patient is not there and most often is unaware. Most doctors truly care about our patients. Plus, there is increased liability in delaying treatment. No doctor certainly wants that.

The War on Doctors

5. Patients are often stuck taking substandard medication because the ones they need are not improved on prior-auth. I am all for generics and cutting costs, but even many generics are now being denied.

While everyone needs to work on cutting costs, it should not be done at the cost of the health of the patient. Doctors are not running amok ordering unnecessary tests to drive up healthcare costs. We need to put more decision-making control back in the hands of the doctors who are actually examining and seeing the patient, not the nameless, faceless ones following their insurance companies' cost-cutting guidelines. Patients deserve better than this.

Insurance companies completely control their formularies and what medications we can choose from. One of the major tasks of doctors is prescribing the correct medications to patients. After discussing options with patients, a treatment plan is devised. It becomes a mere wish as the insurance company overrules that decision. All too often, the medication is not part of an insurance company's formulary and it is too expensive for the patient to pay out-of-pocket. So, who decides these formularies?

As the prescribers, it seems reasonable that doctors would lead the formulary-making process. We are the ones who know what is best for our patients. However, we are usually left out of these decision trees. We may have patients doing well for years on the same medication, but that is no guarantee that they can continue on it. I have too often seen patients forced to change appropriate medications because of formulary changes. To appeal the insurance companies' formulary decisions requires a great amount of time and effort. All too often, this is wasted time and effort. Doctors' frustrations intensify under this system because we feel that we are not able to give the best care to our patients. Most doctors do try to keep healthcare costs in mind, but keeping costs down is not always the best treatment for patients.

Pharmaceutical companies are big drivers in what medications get covered. Much lobbying goes into getting their medication listed. Sure, they have studies showing good outcomes with their products, but they are not always the best outcomes or the only ones with good outcomes. Pharmaceutical companies have a big conflict of interest in helping create formularies because they directly profit from favorable decisions. More head-to-head studies are needed.

Hospitals often devise their own in-house formularies based on cost. This too exerts some influence on insurance formularies. Hospitals see shrinking profits and look for every way to cut costs. This cost reduction derives some benefit from cutting costs on medications used in the hospital setting. Again, there is some conflict of interest here because hospitals increase their profits by deciding what medications they will carry. This is based on dollars, not patient outcomes.

Insurance companies also have a conflict of interest deciding their own formularies. Their profits are maximized when they cover the least costly medications, not necessarily the best medications. I have had prescriptions rejected and been asked to prescribe a completely different class of medication instead. This decision has no basis in patient care or trying to help ease patient suffering but merely in cost savings. Insurance companies have no oversight in devising these formularies. They are completely free to choose and reject any medications they wish.

Much power in making medical decisions has been removed from doctors' hands. The ability to prescribe the best medication for our patients is one example. There is nothing more frustrating for a doctor than to feel that we could give our patients better care but are unable because the insurance companies stand in the way. Further, we know many of the formulary decisions are decided by non-doctors with only cost-savings as the end point. Clinicians need to have more input into these decisions and improved clinical outcomes need to be the goal. We own some of the best medications in the world, but how will they help if we are prevented from using them?

Another area where third parties attack is in the panel of doctors a patient is allowed to choose from. In my area, when the insurance exchanges rolled out, many doctors were suddenly dropped off insurance contracts as insurers narrowed their doctor panels. This was without the knowledge of physicians and without notification. It was not done based on sub-par performance of those doctors. It was done completely to cut

The War on Doctors

costs. I doubt anyone would argue that being deselected from an insurance network "just because" is not a war on doctors. Patients are also being attacked in the process.

I just received a call from a longstanding patient because he learned that we are not in his network under his new insurance plan. However, we always accepted his plan and do not intend to drop it. After closer investigation, his specific plan requires him to use one of several hospital clinics. Everything else is out-of-network. He was not given this information when he signed up for this plan, a plan he is paying for himself. He is not allowed to change plans until October when his next enrollment period rolls out. Insurers are increasingly narrowing their doctor panels.

Last year, in New Jersey, many doctors were suddenly terminated from certain plans they had accepted for many years. This was without prior notice or any discussion. I was not one of those physicians but it caused havoc for doctors and patients alike. It was a play by the insurance company to narrow down the panel to cut costs.

Unfortunately, this narrowing of doctor panels is becoming a frequent occurrence in the healthcare scene. The doctors who are being excluded are not being given any choice or ample notification. Additionally, the doctors being deselected are not being chosen by quality criteria. The driving force is reducing costs, which thereby increases insurance company profits. Patients should be allowed to have the highest care, not bargain basement discounts.

People are clamoring for patients to be empowered consumers, to advocate for themselves and take a greater role in their own medical decision-making. How is that even possible when they are denied access to the doctors they want to treat them? Many patients are forced to leave doctors who they feel comfortable with and who have treated them for years.

Why should patients be allowed to see the doctors they want?

- The doctor-patient relationship is essential for good outcomes. A patient is not going to follow the advice of a doctor they do not trust. Likewise, doctors need to trust that patients are giving them accurate information.
- Patients were promised that under the ACA they would be allowed to keep their doctors. Promises should be kept.
- Patients are now paying an increasing amount into their own health insurance coverage. They should be allowed to choose the doctor that provides them medical care. It is unjustifiable that they are forced to pay their own premiums and then deny them access to the care that they want.
- Only patients and the doctors should determine what is in the best medical interests for each individual patient. Third parties, such as insurance companies, need to stop intruding into this relationship and overturning health care decisions. This is harming patients.

As the ACA becomes more deeply entrenched, patients are footing more of their healthcare expenses. As the consumers of these products, they should have choices of where they receive their care. If a person wants to eat dinner out, they can spend their money at any restaurant of their choosing. When they purchase a car, there are no limits on where they can shop. Why is a patient's health and wellbeing valued at less than these services? It will change only if doctors demand to stay in network with insurance plans. Patients need to stand up and demand options.

Why are third parties at war with doctors anyway?

In my mind, the answer is very simple: corporate greed. These third party insurance companies work hard to decrease reimbursements to doctors and maximize their own profits. The greed of corporate players is perhaps the most powerful warring faction against doctors and it is destroying our healthcare system.

The War on Doctors

In 2013, the CEO of Aetna earned $33.7 million dollars. The average health insurance CEO salary was over $10 million in that same time period. While many will say that is capitalism at work, I really wonder, as I fight to get another MRI covered for a patient, how many MRIs were denied to generate that kind of salary? The year 2014 saw great increases in member enrollment in insurance plans under the ACA. Profits for these plans jumped up tens of millions of dollars.

My patients are suffering. They cannot afford the premiums they are now forced to pay, often against their will. They cannot afford the high deductibles most of these plans now carry. I have seen patients decide between two needed medications and which of their family members was the sickest to take to the doctor. They could not afford both.

Every day, I see more and more diagnostic tests and procedures being denied by insurance companies. I spend hours a week fighting these denials. Most insurance companies have now limited their formularies to exclusively generics. Even so, the expensive generics, such as life-saving asthma inhalers, are being denied.

My patients are struggling to afford their healthcare. Many are ending up having bad medical consequences because they cannot afford to get the medical care that they need. I have sent more than one asthmatic patient to the ER who had a severe exacerbation of their disease because their inhaler was too expensive and no longer covered by their insurance plan. While patients are struggling to get care, the insurance companies are making obscene profits. The CEOs of these companies make salaries like few other industries. Surely, a financial conflict of interest must exist to deny medical care. Yet, there is no one regulating the insurance companies. They hold free reign in what they approve and disallow. They ignore the medical advice doctors give their own patients and override their decisions. Yet, they are protected from liability.

Linda Girgis

As more and more care is denied, the quality of our entire healthcare system is degraded. When I see a patient for a 15-minute visit and then spend days trying to get their medication approved, our priorities have been misplaced. When the insurance company overrides my clinical acumen based on their predetermined guidelines, medicine and science are tossed out the window to contain costs. There needs to be a collaborative effort to reduce healthcare spending, but not at the cost of the wellbeing of patients.

In our system, patients are now seen as consumers. While getting them to be advocates for themselves is a great thing, their humanity is getting lost in the process. Having a hip replacement is not the same as shopping for a set of kitchen knives at Wal-Mart. They need to be respected as more than just consumers. So many people talk about Big Data these days. Patients are more than just their medical information. They are real people with real needs, and no two of them are exactly alike.

Corporate greed, especially of health insurance companies, is destroying our healthcare system and the medical wellbeing of patients everywhere. We need to put the person back in the patient and get corporate decisions out of the exam room. Medical decisions need to be made based on the best interests of each individual patient, whether they fit into the insurance companies' clinical pathways or not. We need to consider cost, but not at the expense of the patient. Doctors' decisions serve the best interests of our patients and we need to be able to practice medicine, not comply with regulations. Do we really want bargain basement medicine or is it time to restore the US healthcare system back to the best?

Third parties have overstepped their boundaries in the treatment of patients. They practice medicine without medical licenses and restrict what care patients are allowed to receive. Their decisions are made without any direct knowledge of patients and without ever performing physical exams. Yet, their decisions are law and the treating doctor's hands are all too often tied by this system. Isn't it time to get these money-hungry warmongers to stop practicing medicine? Do patients want to be medically treated by a greedy organization? Or do we want doctors helping us decide the best medical options for us based on direct patient knowledge and physical exams?

Chapter 3 Governmental Takeover of Medicine

Last week, a patient became upset at my receptionist for being required to sign too many forms. As any patient knows, there are certain forms that must be signed to protect his/her privacy. The federal Health Insurance Portability and Accountability Act, also known as HIPAA, passed in 1996 and requires doctors and healthcare providers to explain to a patient their rights under this act. Most facilities provide patients a form to read explaining these rights and the patients are asked to sign that it was provided to them and they read it. Well, this patient just refused to sign it and asked what would happen. Unfortunately, without this signature, we cannot submit insurance charges on the patients' behalf. This patient finally relented and signed when he realized he would have to pay and submit the charges on his own. While protecting patients' privacy is a good goal, it seems lately the government has run amok with issuing their mandates. We now have MU, PQRS, PCMH, MACRA, and a whole alphabet soup of regulations we must submit to. When will doctors find enough time to treat patients with this slew of new laws? Do we really want our politicians controlling what happens between the doctor and the patient in the exam rooms across the US?

Healthcare spending in the US is one of the largest expenditures in our country. For this reason, everyone wants to grab a piece or the pie, or at least control how healthcare dollars are being spent. Mandates about our healthcare system flow out of the halls of our government like never before. But enough mandates! Do we really want politicians making medical decisions for us? Or should doctors be able to practice medicine and do right for our patients? It all too often feels like Big Brother is in the exam room along with me, and I need to obtain his permission before ordering tests or prescribing medications.

Doctors, for the most part, feel that we no longer have much control over the direction the healthcare system is headed. In fact, 44% of doctors polled on SERMO (the largest social media network exclusive to physicians) responded that they have very little control over healthcare policy. On the front lines, doctors need to heed insurance company guidelines to get certain tests performed. This happens even when it is clear that a patient has departed from an expected clinical course. The decision is left in the hands of a non-medical, or medical if it is raised to peer review, person. This person has never seen, examined, or even spoken with my patient. Sometimes, they do read my encounter notes. But most often, the decision is determined based on an ICD-9 code. Patients are indeed now numbers to private and government insurers.

Doctors can no longer keep a medical record to be able to follow the patient's clinical course. The government stepped in and made up the Meaningful Use program, which began its existence with the passage of the HITECH Act in 2009. Now, we must enter "metrics" (as the government calls them) into the patients' charts. While some may think this a wise idea, I can guarantee they have never actually undertaken the task while evaluating and treating patients in real-time. It is a bottleneck in the practice's workflow, from the receptionist who has to ask the patient's race and email address (even when the patient doesn't want to give it) to the medical assistant who needs to document many metrics into the patient chart to keep us compliant with meaningful use requirements. Patients don't like it either. It annoys them when the doctor and other staff spend the time looking at the computer instead of them. Does anyone not treating patients actually get this?

The PCM (patient-centered medical home) is another vacuum of time waste. The paperwork burden to be certified can kill a practice. To submit all the required screenshots for certification required dedicating one of my staff full-time to the task for weeks to complete. Small practices do not have IT departments or extra hands on deck.

Now the recent passage of the MACRA bill will dump more regulatory burdens onto doctors. People rejoice in the demise of the SGR. But at what cost? Our payment models are now mandated by federal law. Does anyone see how this can possibly be a good thing? The same people who gave us the SGR that took years to repeal now have a bigger control over the healthcare system.

Currently, it seems like new regulations are being made for doctors every day. While keeping up with these new mandates is burdensome for everyone, it is causing havoc on small practices. Unlike larger groups or hospitals, we just do not have the staff to implement all these changes. Nor can we afford it even if we wanted it. While many proclaim these new requirements, such as Meaningful Use, NCQA, e-prescribing, etc., are going to improve clinical outcomes, many doctors are just not seeing that reality.

How are increasing mandates harmful?

- Doctors need to spend increasing time keeping up with these mandates. Unfortunately, we cannot do everything at the same time so we need to find this time somewhere. Often, the only place left is the time we spend with patients. Patient diseases are becoming more complex and new treatments are proliferating. Is it better for a doctor to spend time learning the latest treatment options that can be offered to a patient, or to use that time learning which box to check so our metrics are adequately captured by the regulators?
- When these regulations become standard, often the thinking process goes out the window. For example, prior authorizations for diagnostic tests and medications are often decided by people who are not physicians and are just following guidelines. Even when doctors appeal and state the reason why the patient needs a certain procedure or medication, it is often arbitrarily denied. Surely, some clinical reasoning should go into denials for services a doctor feels necessary for their patients. Additionally, doctors have been speaking up against Meaningful Use mandates. Many of us don't feel the EHR technology is there yet to be clinically useful. Yet, there are metrics in place that we need to record to prove we are using it meaningfully. This disconnect is also hazardous. Doctors need to be data entry clerks to record metrics that we don't feel are beneficial to our patients. Is it better if doctors decide how to use their EHR for the best patient care?

The War on Doctors

- Implementing the necessary practice changes to keep in compliance is costly. Physicians are probably the only profession that does not receive cost of living increases to our salaries. Our reimbursements are shrinking and/or stagnating. Overhead costs are soaring. It is already very difficult financially to keep our doors open. Yet, this added burden is being cast around our necks. Isn't it better for doctors to invest in new services and technology for patient care rather than investing in metrics recording for insurance companies?
- In small practices, staff needs to take on the role of doing this additional work. They too are only human and can do so much. They need to take time away from other tasks to accomplish the requirements set forth. This too is time taken away from patients. Wouldn't it be better for the staff in a doctor's office to concentrate on patients?

While data can be a good thing, when it goes overboard it can have the opposite effect of what was intended. We all want improved clinical outcomes and the spirit of some of these requirements is not all bad. When the regulations become the primary goal, patient care will suffer. It is time to put the patient back in the spotlight. They are the ones we are all working for. It is time to make regulations that are clinically useful and focus on the patient. Maybe it is time to put doctors in charge of that task rather than executives and politicians.

A good example of what happens when the government intrudes into mandating healthcare was its attempt to budget Medicare. The Balanced Budget Act, passed in 1997 by Congress, adopted the SGR (Sustainable Growth Rate), which aimed to control federal healthcare spending. Basically, the SGR formula aims to keep the total increase in Medicare reimbursements to physicians from exceeding the change in GDP (Gross Domestic Product).

However, since its inception, the cost of reimbursing healthcare services rose faster than the increase in GDP. In order to prevent Medicare recipients from going without care, Congress has fallen into the convention of passing temporary short-term fixes to the SGR formula. In fact, Congress has passed 17 such stopgap fixes since the onset of this legislation.

On March 26, 2015, the House passed the HR2/SGR Repeal bill that would repeal the SGR formula by a substantial majority. Many proclaim this to be a rare bipartisan victory. This bill was passed by the Senate in April and signed into law a day later by President Obama.

Many people look at this bill and see that it will repeal the ill-fated SGR formula and throw their support behind it. However, this bill consists of 250 pages, all written in legal language. People miss many of the other actions hidden in this Trojan horse bill. When reviewed in totality, its impact on the future of healthcare is quite adverse.

One of the measures of this bill would be to turn away from traditional fee-for-service payments to providers and move to outcome-based ones. For example, as a physician, I would get paid depending on whether a patient chose to heed my advice, as well as the care I provide. Yet, the full burden falls on me as the provider of the service. The patient bears no responsibility for making unhealthy lifestyle choices.

While the proponents proclaim that this will lead to improved clinical outcomes, they are blinded to the whole picture. Doctors cannot afford to practice uncompensated. Overhead costs soar and our salaries have remained stagnant for the past decade. What will likely happen is that doctors will deselect the more non-compliant and complex patients. Additionally, many doctors will opt out of Medicare completely.

Where will those Medicare patients receive care? It is estimated that in the US, approximately 8,000 people turn 65 years old every day.

The government should ensure healthcare for our nation's elderly and not drive doctors out of business and force others to opt out. Doctors should be reimbursed for the extra work we give these patients, many of whom have numerous medical problems and will have poor outcomes no matter what we do to help them.

The War on Doctors

But the government is at war with doctors. Politicians do not want us to practice independently, and there is a strong push to herd us all into these large groups. This will help the government gain more control over us. The healthcare industry represents big money to these politicians. Their push is not about creating a better healthcare system, but rather winning control of the finances. To do that, we need to be yoked with this burdensome chain of mandates. Doctors in small practices are drowning in the flood of these useless legal requirements. Many people theorize that this is the first step to single-payer government-controlled health insurance. If we look at the rollout of the ACA and the insurance exchange program, there appears to be some truth in that. Do we really want the government in charge of our health? Look at how they managed our economy and the ill-fated SGR program before answering. Is there any reason at all that politicians should be defining what constitutes good health outcomes? Just remember that Congress is exempt from the ACA insurance exchanges and members are insured by their own special coverage. Should a doctor have to justify why they are treating a patient in a certain way to a governmental entity? There are cases of billing abuse and fraud out there. Doctors think those guilty parties should be prosecuted to the full extent of the law. We just think there are too many politicians and governmental employees in the exam room trying to steal the reins of medical decision making. Isn't it time that the doctor and patient should be left alone and make these decisions together, without forced regulations from unseen and uncaring parties?

It is hard to keep up with all these new regulations. However, as doctors, we have to or face dire consequences for not complying. People have full-time jobs in healthcare policy and regulation. Doctors need to learn it in between patients. How much money does it cost to regulate healthcare so much? Does anyone suppose it may actually save money just to let doctors practice medicine?

Chapter 4 Minimizing the Profession: Who Needs Doctors?

The use of nurse practitioners and physician assistants continues to rise exponentially. Are they needed in medicine? Yes, they certainly are an important part of the healthcare system and I love the ones I collaborate with. They are not doctors, nor will they ever be doctors. We are trained differently and possess a different skill set. There seems to be a push recently to fill the shortage of physicians with mid-level providers. This will hurt us all. While mid-levels are becoming more important in our healthcare system, it is important that we do not blur the lines of differences between us.

For years, experts have predicted a physician shortage, especially in the primary care fields. Little has been done to increase the number of physicians choosing to pursue these specialties or increase the number of doctors to fill the gap. Rather, some are calling for mid-level providers to step up and fill this deficiency. While mid-levels can greatly assist and are much-needed in primary care, they are still not physicians and will not fill the gap. While they can work unsupervised in some states, in others they can only work under a physician's supervision.

Why Mid-Levels Will Not Fill The Primary Care Gap

- Their training is different. They are educated and trained to be mid-levels. Doctors are educated and trained to be doctors. They are not interchangeable. They are a great asset, but they are not trained to be doctors and should not be used to replace doctors.
- Many patients prefer being treated by physicians. While I have nothing against a patient who would rather see a mid-level provider than me, the patient should have enough options to be able to choose whom they would like to see. They should not be forced to be treated by a mid-level because there are just not any physicians available for them. In the final analysis, we are all

working for good outcomes for the patients and helping them be their own advocates.

- Mid-levels are not as well-trained to treat high-risk patients. Many people have stated that the increased number of mid-levels will result in doctors seeing the high-risk patients. However, as the population ages, so does the number of high-risk patients. There will be many more complicated patients resulting from increasing age, the rising incidences of obesity, diabetes mellitus and other chronic diseases. The number of physicians must increase to match these needs.
- Mid-levels still need to call on physicians when they have questions. While they can see and treat patients, in some states without supervision, they still need doctors available as backup. Doctors are already overwhelmed by the increasing number of patients and demands being placed on us. Not all of us have any time left to supervision the growing number of mid-levels now practicing.

While mid-levels can help ease the looming physician shortage, they are not going to fill the void. More doctors are still going to be needed. As more patients are being insured under the ACA, more doctors need to be available. To provide the highest quality care, a team approach needs to be taken. Mid-levels provide a valuable service to medicine and are highly competent to treat many medical conditions. However, they still cannot replace doctors. As more and more patients become insured, as patients age and more complex medical problems arise, we are still going to need more physicians. Yet, the number of physicians being educated and trained has not increased very much in recent years. While an individual doctor may feel overwhelmed and overworked by the shortage, the true crisis is the lack of access. This will be felt most by the ones we are all trying to help: the patient.

The media is full of articles of mid-level practitioners filling the void that the physician shortage is creating. Yes, they are needed and can help alleviate the problem. But we need to remember the difference between them and doctors. Only doctors can be doctors. As the population ages, we are going to need more doctors.

Also very evident in the media are articles about doctors being replaced by technology. Some theorize that computers and robots will take over the tasks that doctors perform. Instead of getting the human touch by your personal physician, the supercomputer Watson will alleviate your ailments. Robots will operate on you. It sounds like something right off *Star Trek* or *The Jetsons*.

An article in the *New York Times* talks about how technology possesses an enormous potential in healthcare. It cites as evidence the plethora of fitness trackers now available on the market. This article points to a conference held in San Francisco where a third of the attendees agreed with speaker, Dr. Vivek Wadhwa, when he said that he would rather be treated by a doctor with artificial rather than human intelligence. This article goes on to list several innovative data collecting devices that are being made available. Some of them were no longer being used because they failed to show improved outcomes. [1] Technology and innovation are absolutely essential in medicine. We need to keep driving new ideas and new resources to improve patient care. These devices cannot replace doctors either. Doctors are still very much essential in analyzing the data and making inferences on how it affects health. A fitness tracker can potentially change someone's life. Unless you know what to do with the data collected from it, you are deriving no benefit. Technology and innovation are good but unless you marry them to the experts (doctors) that know how to use them, they will become rather useless. Doctors who fail to adapt innovation and technology are committing wrongs as well. Patients deserve the most advanced medical treatments, delivered by the hands of the most skilled.

An article in the *Wall Street Journal* tells us that IBM's supercomputer Watson will one day take the place of doctors. According to the author, the digitalization of records makes this a "foregone conclusion." He states that computers are better able to store, cross-reference, and retrieve data than the human brain ever will be. I absolutely agree with this. Medicine is so much more than just data. [2] Will Watson know that my patient has a secret Dorito's obsession and that is why her blood pressure is always high? Will Watson be able to ascertain that my patient's spouse was just laid off from work and that is why she is not sleeping at night? There will always be the need for the human touch in medicine. Watson and all the supercomputers in the world are just tools available for use by man to improve our profession.

Another article in *Fortune* explains how technology will replace 80% of what doctors are currently doing. According to the writer of this article, healthcare is currently about the "practice of medicine" and not the "science of medicine." Doctors apparently only practice with half-remembered and obsolete lessons learned in medical school. Additionally, according to the author, our practice is full of cognitive and recency biases and other human errors. It was postulated that healthcare should be data-driven and less about "trial and error." The conclusion of this article is that data will improve care, reduce costs, and reduce physician work- loads. This article explains how computers do better than doctors by using sensors and data collection and then performing analytics. Furthermore, "Computers are better at organizing and recalling complex information than a hotshot Harvard MD. They're also better at integrating and balancing considerations of patient symptoms, history, demeanor, environmental factors, and population management guidelines than the average physician. Besides, 50% of MDs are below average! Computers also have much lower error rates. Shouldn't we take advantage of that when it comes to our health?" But, it also suggests that this technology will not happen overnight but rather in baby steps (wouldn't you call that trial and error that the author so much opposes?). [3]

I find much wrong with this article. Firstly, doctors do practice science every day. We are not prescribing medicine based on whims or our mood of the day. There is a large body of knowledge that exists called evidence-based medicine. This is medicine that has been studied and proven to be beneficial. This is the science, not a set of data points. Additionally, doctors are required to continue learning throughout our careers. We need to prove it or we cannot be licensed to practice medicine. The author's remark that we are practicing on half-remembered and obsolete information we learned in medical school is factually incorrect, and biased in my opinion. The author states that 50% of doctors are below average. If you look at the average of anything, 50% will be above average and 50% below average. In computer productivity, there will be 50% above the average and 50% below. This is just the definition of averages that the author is trying to toy with to make doctors appear substandard. However, this article is a clear example of how doctors are being minimized and increasingly seen as expendable. Do we need technology and better computers in medicine? Absolutely, and I dream of a computer that would be able to aid me in clinical diagnostics. To imagine a computer that can do this without the human hand is ludicrous. Only an expert should be at the keyboard of this medical supercomputer highway.

In the *Washington Post,* a theory postulated by Farhad Manjoo about the future of medicine is discussed. He feels that robots will take over medicine—and not just the lowest technological jobs—but the most highly specialized ones as well. Apparently, the author feels that most doctors lack empathy although they are good at science. He states, "But then, we're not sitting in that room wrapped in a garment made of the finest recycled sandpaper because we were hoping for a good conversation. We're there because we're sick, or worried we might be sick, and we're hoping this arrogant, hurried, credentialed genius can tell us what's wrong. We go to doctors not because they're great empaths, but because we're hoping medical school has made them into the closest thing the human race has developed to robots." According to Manjoo's theory, robots are built to do surgery. He feels that robots will take over healthcare by specializing. The author, however, thinks that robots will undermine primary care long before the specialties. According to the author, the people in the health care system that are good at talking to patients are the nurses. His vision is that the nurse can converse well with the patient and put information into the computer and by doing so, they will be given the correct diagnosis or medication the patient needs. The nurse can then refer the patient to the correct specialist based on the computer-generated opinion. They will do so at less expense than doctors and are better at talking to patients. [4] So, who needs doctors?

This article is full of biases against doctors, who are referred to as arrogant, hurried, type-A personalities who possess poor communication skills. The author apparently only sees doctors because they are the closest thing to a robot that can be human. In my mind, it is never good

The War on Doctors

to generalize about any group of people: you will always be wrong at some point. The fact that the author sees nurses as being able to do a better job than doctors is telling. I love nurses and have a great relationship with the ones I work with. I could not do my job without them. However, they are not doctors. They are not all friendly either. I had the personal experience of dealing with Nurse Ratchet when I underwent a medical test. Some of them are arrogant and some are quite Type-A and aggressive. So, perhaps the author should have suggested that only nice people with good communication skills should man the robot? But, at the end of the day, we need everyone in the healthcare system. Robotics have already made great achievements in certain types of surgery. They cannot do it without the guidance of expert surgical hands. I honestly hope we see more innovation roll out in robotics and technology and I do hope it can do some of my work. We cannot separate the importance of anyone in the system: doctors, nurses, technicians, etc. We all play a very important and vital role in the lives of our patients.

The Atlantic carried a story about a robot, IBM's Watson being used at Memorial Sloan-Kettering to learn to make diagnoses and treatment recommendations. The preface of this article again asks if doctors are really necessary. According to this article, Watson can process up to 60 million pages per second. just as Watson improved at playing *Jeopardy,* it is expected to improve at diagnosing medical problems and determining ways to treat them the more that it interacts with patient cases. It also can express if it has doubts by assigning a level of confidence to each recommendation that it makes. Memorial Sloan-Kettering has stepped in as a sort of tutor to Watson. The hospital is feeding it real clinical cases and teaching how to make sense of this medical information. It is felt that this tool can be very helpful in a field such as oncology because of all the new information coming out and all the subtleties around cancer care. Memorial Sloan-Kettering is not the lone hospital trying to shape Watson into an effective clinical tool. The Cleveland Clinic is trying to develop Watson into a training tool for young physicians and perhaps later as a bedside tool. Silicon Valley is entering the foray as well. Many are scrambling to devise this technology to be usable in the healthcare setting.[5]

While this article does seem to make it clear that Watson is a tool to be used by human doctor hands, it does quote a venture capitalist as saying that computers and robots will replace four out of five physicians in the near future. Again, this technology and innovation is great and possesses a huge potential to disrupt the healthcare field; do we really want to eliminate the human touch and be treated by machines?

There are many other references projecting the opinion that doctors are replaceable by computers and robots. This opinion is at war with doctors by minimizing our skills and the human art of medicine. Sure, this technology and innovation will disrupt healthcare hopefully for the better. Do we want that to be all there is between us and the cure of a disease? Despite what many of the writers stated, there are still plenty of doctors full of empathy. Do you want a computer generated print out telling you what you need to know? Or do you want a person to feel the pain you are in, to understand you are suffering? A computer or robot does not own shoulders you can cry on. Very often, that is all my patients need. No algorithm can be programmed to develop this; it is human emotion. Medical treatment devoid of human emotion is cruel. Our patients need empathy and care. Do I want to see Watson and other innovations succeed? Yes, but they should never replace the human factor. We need to care about our patients on an emotional level. Sometimes a hug is all that is needed. Are doctors replaceable? Only if you want cold-hearted assembly-line medicine.

1- http://www.nytimes.com/2014/09/21/sunday-review/high-tech-health-care-useful-to-a-point.html?_r=0
2- http://blogs.wsj.com/experts/2014/06/10/will-computers-replace-doctors/
3- http://fortune.com/2012/12/04/technology-will-replace-80-of-what-doctors-do/
4- http://www.washingtonpost.com/blogs/ezra-klein/post/how-robots-will-replace-doctors/2011/08/25/gIQASA17AL_blog.html
5- http://www.theatlantic.com/magazine/archive/2013/03/the-robot-will-see-you-now/309216/

Chapter 5 Angry Patients

Patients are angry, and who can blame them? They are being crushed by the system and turning their frustrations on doctors. They are forced to pay for premiums they may not want to under the ACA (commonly known as Obamacare), and after paying these premiums, all too often, they have high deductibles they must meet before their insurance plan will cover anything. To make the whole situation worse, insurance companies narrowed panels of doctors from which patients can choose and have also decreased formulary coverage. In essence, patients are now paying more and receiving fewer services and fewer choices. This does not even factor in physician shortages and lack of access.

Patients often direct their anger at doctors. Sure, some of it may be justified. But, the doctors frequently are trapped in the middle between the battles of the patients and the insurance companies. Commonly, some of the wrath is tossed our way. The expectation is there that we can force the insurance company to cover things that they have refused the patient. No, we cannot. There is no one more frustrated about this situation than doctors. We spend hours just trying to get approvals for tests and medications we believe our patients need. This anger erodes trust both ways.

Here is one example of the distrust in doctors. I received this email in response to an article I published regarding vaccines. Sure, it is not talking about the subject of denied care. However, it does show the disdain that many people now have for doctors.

> "I read your recent article concerning your "war" with non-vax parents. I want you to know, parents are aware doctors believe they know best. However, the statistics show otherwise. Doctor's mistakes are now the third leading cause of death in our country. Our children are sicker than ever before, 54% of them have a chronic illness. We also have the highest infant mortality rates in the developed world. As a parent, it is my right to choose to inject my child with pharmaceutical poison or not. I choose not. In my

search for a pediatrician, I found several who refused to see my perfectly healthy and neurotypical children for check-ups...so, do you know what I did? I found a doctor who would...and he receives MY money. Although, visits are never needed—because my kids are never sick, not mentally or physically. We aren't stupid; this is what all of us are doing. Doctors who bully and disrespect a parent's right to choose...are not hurting us; they are hurting their own pocket books. So, continue your war, before long, there won't be anyone left to fight, as, word is spreading like wild fire."

Patients are losing trust in doctors. This is a bad thing. A patient who does not trust their doctor is not going to listen to their advice. In my mind, the doctor-patient relationship is sacrosanct. There is no relationship where the bond of trust should be so strong, outside of matrimony. As physicians, patients rely on us to help them make life-saving decisions. We need patients to be honest with us so that we can give the highest quality medical advice. Yet, there has been an erosion in this relationship over recent years. Doctors are no longer held in such high esteem as they were decades ago. They feel we don't listen to their concerns anymore and don't care what they want or need.

Why has the public lost trust in doctors?
- Third parties are often making decisions. For example, they dictate their own formularies, and we often have our hands tied as to what medications we can prescribe. I often have patients ask me for the "strong Stuff." They don't realize that doctors are limited in prescribing habits, and we are not withholding the Best medications. We are the ones in direct contact with the patient.
- Outlier doctors have been gaming the system. Most doctors truly put patients' care first, before profit. But, there are a few who inappropriately use their medical degrees for profit. Just look at Dr. Oz trying to get rich promoting weight loss products with no proven benefit. These doctors make us all look bad.
- There are many mandates imposed on us that affect patient care. One example is meaningful use. Doctors now have to document many metrics, inputting data into our EHR systems, in order to meet requirements. Patients take this lack of eye-to-eye contact

as a sign that we are more interested in their digital record than them. They feel we are no longer listening to them. They don't realize that we don't want to be doing this. It has been opposed on us from on high, and we will be penalized if we don't.

- HMO's have greatly cut reimbursements to doctors. In order for practices to stay afloat financially, we have to see more patients. We need to find more and more room to see these extra patients if we want to stay afloat. Patients feel this and take it as an indication that we are pushing them through for profit and don't care about them.
- Media tends to portray doctors in a bad light. There are big stories about the pill mill doctors and those arrested for fraud or harassment. There are so many more amazing stories of heroic doctors around than the bad apples. But the press does not give them attention. People rather see the bad than the good. This too tends to paint us all in a negative light.

  Medical diseases are becoming more complex, and people are living longer. There has never been a time where patients need to trust their doctors more. All doctors need to remember their oath and put the patient back in center focus. We all need to take a stand against those doctors who are abusing the system for their own gain. Patients need to learn that the vast majority us care about our patients and have their best interests in mind. We all need to become a team again. Patients need to regain our trust, and our profession needs to re-establish its integrity.

While most patients still trust us, those that don't go to war with us. This afternoon, a patient came to his appointment two and a half hours late, after we closed. The staff was checking messages and I was sending refills before I left. While the rush to leave for the day ensued, this patient walked in and demanded to be seen. My receptionist explained that he was more than two hours late and the office was closed. He demanded to be seen and he knew I was still in the office. But, my daughter was waiting for me to pick her up. Doctors have families too, lives outside the office. Patients who make unreasonable demands beat us down.

Frequently, the doctor is trapped in the middle between angry patients and their insurance battles. The blame is cast upon us when their tests get denied or they cannot get their desired medication because of their insurance company's formularies. Doctors understand that, we really do.

Linda Girgis

In fact, most of the days of a primary care doctor is spent in this war. We want to give you what you want but, contrary to many patients' beliefs, we cannot force the insurance company to cover what they don't want to. Doctors are not hiding in their offices playing "Angry Birds" with their patients' lives. We don't order tests that later get denied just for the joy of it. We spend hours on this and are more frustrated than anyone else. If you are frustrated about one denial, imagine five or six every day, day in and day out. We understand why patients get angry but when that anger is turned on us, it wrecks the bond we formed. Doctors and patients are on the same team. The only way to achieve victory is when we realize this and work together.

While doctors all see patients who are upset or angry, it sometimes goes to the extremes. There are occasions when doctors even face violence when we are treating patients. The murder of Dr. Michael Davidson, a cardiac surgeon at Brigham and Women's Hospital, has saddened and horrified us all. He was shot to death while on duty at his workplace on January 20, 2015 by the disgruntled son of a deceased patient. As time passes, we hear all the stories of what a remarkable doctor he was and feel the loss in our medical community.

However, his death has further struck a chord with many of us. Doctors are all thinking, "That could have been me," as we recall aggressive and hostile patients we have encountered in the past. Few doctors have never had a patient that they were genuinely afraid of or been threatened by. The more years we practice, the more such stories we can tell.

The worst I personally encountered was a patient I refused to give a prescription of a controlled substance because I felt that she was abusing it. She went home, called my staff, and told them to get out of the way because she was coming back to kill me. She ended up with 6 months of probation and a permanent restraining order against me. I spent many months looking over my shoulder.

It is especially difficult for our emergency room colleagues who have no choice which patients they must treat. They have to see every patient that walks through the doors. Many of them have been victims of violence and aggression. Yet, if these same patients walk through those doors again, there is no choice but to treat them again.

The War on Doctors

While we understand that patients are often not at their best when they see us, there are limits to what behavior is tolerable. Some patients threaten to sue us if they don't get what they want. Others become verbally abusive and still others threaten physical violence. Doctors should never be demanded to prescribe medicine they judge inappropriate out of fear of their lives or medical licenses.

The example of Dr. Davidson should serve as an example to us all of the extremes disgruntled patients can go to when they are not happy. Too many doctors feel they have no control over these situations and their employers often dictate that they must continue to treat these patients. Many are lax in protecting doctors and healthcare workers because a murder such as this is just so unbelievable. We need to all be on alert. As more patients become disgruntled in our current healthcare system, hostilities rise. A doctor, or anyone else for that matter, should not be forced to treat or deal with someone they are fearful of.

Doctors also need more training on managing explosive situations in the exam room. Usually, we are totally focused on the patient's medical condition. We need to have protocols in place when we feel a patient is getting aggressive. It is never wrong to call the police if we feel threatened. For the most part, the police are very sympathetic to our concerns.

No doctor should ever be the victim of violence by patients or their families. Patients may not like our decisions and this is their right. But it is never justified to take out their frustrations in violent and hostile ways. If someone is unhappy with a doctor, go find a new one. If someone feels they were harmed by the actions of a doctor, there is a tort system in place to discuss their concerns. We need to protect those on the front lines saving lives. Society needs their skills and they are irreplaceable. The world lost a great lifesaver and man in Dr. Davidson. We should all strive to make sure that this never happens again.

It happens too often recently that a patient will arrive for a visit and be shocked that they owe a deductible. Some will become rude to the staff and even become aggressive. But they are taking their wrath out on the wrong people. Doctors do not determine what a patient's deductible is. This is completely decided by the insurance company and the patient should be aware of the plan they signed up for. Some of them expect us to not collect the deductible, as if doctors should work for free and they are entitled to medical service at no cost. Unfortunately, this is the system we are all working in. Not only can I not afford to toil for free, it is against the law for me to do so. According to federal anti-kickback laws, writing off any payment would be viewed as a kick-back to the patient for choosing me to provide medical services to them. Not only am I not willing to work for free, I am totally opposed to going to jail or being fined for any patient who requests my enslavement to them. Yes, they are angry, but they wage their war on doctors, who literally have no control over this aspect of the system. I understand where their anger comes from, but it needs to be directed where it can effect some change—the insurance companies.

I was sitting listening to a patient's litany of offenses another doctor committed against her. From her description, her previous doctor must have been named Dr. Satan. While she did have some valid concerns, I knew that she would do the same against me if the situation ever arose. Of course, there are bad doctors practicing medicine. But there are some who just possess a personality that clashes with a given patient. My advice to patients is that they should never be treated by a doctor that they are uncomfortable around. It doesn't mean that there is anything bad about a given doctor or about the patient. It is just a mismatch in personalities and that is OK because this is reality. I say the same about me. If they don't feel confident in my advice, I encourage them to seek out other opinions. Again, there is nothing wrong with being angry. But it should be directed at the right party and a patient should not leave themselves in the hands of a doctor they are angry with. This only creates animosity and a wedge in the therapeutic relationship. The fact that this patient was angry at another physician did indeed set up a barrier in her care. For one thing, it consumed a good portion of the office visit. For another, I developed a certain distrust of her. Trust needs to go both ways between the patient and the doctor to have a truly beneficial therapeutic relationship.

The War on Doctors

A patient was upset that she was required to pay a deductible for two of her office visits. She was not a poor person; both she and her husband work at good jobs. It wasn't that she couldn't afford to pay the deductible. She just felt that it was unfair that she was expected to pay anything. If I write off a deductible, I am actually guilty of providing a kickback for my services. Basically, it is against federal law for me to reduce fees to my patients. Besides, why should doctors be expected to work for free? If she did not pay the deductible, I would not be paid anything. Despite much protest, we collected the payment. Later, her husband came and demanded the money back. I wondered if he does that after he fills his car with gas or buys his groceries at the supermarket. The situation became quite ugly and he threatened to call the police and have me arrested for stealing their money. We advised him to call his insurance company to understand the terms of his insurance coverage.

Patients are becoming increasingly fed up with the system. Who bears the blame? It is often the doctor because we are the only ones face-to-face with the patient. If a diagnostic test is denied, the patient is sent a letter by their insurance company. Good luck if they can reach a living person at the insurance company to get any details about the denial. Hold times are typically over 30 minutes but can sometimes be over an hour. Unable to reach the responsible person, the patient vents at us. We understand. However, we probably are much more frustrated because we deal with this many times a day. When the insurance company decides benefits, I am not given any say into this. If you have a deductible, that is completely between you and your insurance company. Lately, deductibles have sky-rocketed. I agree that it is a burden but I am not the one that can fix it. There are many patients angry about the rising out-of-pocket expenses, yet everyone keeps paying them. It will only change with group action and when everyone speaks up.

In my area, we are seeing a rising incidence of heroin addiction. Many of these patients started off by being addicted to opioid pain medications. We are seeing more patients requesting these medications inappropriately. They get angry when they are refused. Doctors across the country are feeling this. As physicians, we have all been faced with patients inappropriately looking for prescriptions for controlled substances. Some are looking to abuse them and some to divert them for profit. It is often hard to distinguish when a patient truly needs these medications or when they are just "drug-seeking." More experienced doctors have a better sense of which patients are which. Drug-seeking patients often play on our emotions because they know we generally care about patients and may have difficulty turning down a request for opioids from someone in supposed pain. For years, patients have used many ruses to access these medications. Many of them "doctor shop," use several pharmacies, or frequent various emergency rooms, making it difficult to track their prescriptions. It's much harder for a doctor to turn down a request from a new patient in acute pain than from one the doctor knows well and doubts. Having so many controlled substances available and sold on the streets has led to an increase in prescription drug dependency. These patients have a hard time breaking these addictions and often can only stop with help from special rehab programs. It has led to a further resurgence of IV heroin addiction and opioid deaths in many areas. As the states have tightened controlled substance prescriptions, they have become less available for diversion and are now a gateway drug to heroin—which is cheaper than prescribed medications. I am seeing teens in my practice addicted to IV heroin, a habit that started by raiding parents' or relatives' medicine cabinets. It has never been more imperative for doctors to step up and do their part in stopping the supply of inappropriate substances being available for diversion.

This war is particularly wearing on physicians. We don't want to deny patients in need but we also don't want to fuel anyone's addiction. Throw angry patients into the mix and it gets unbearable at times. This war is not just aimed at doctors, but all workers in the healthcare industry.

According to an article published by the CDC, there are more than 5 million workers in US hospitals in a wide variety of occupations. Some recent data shows that hospital workers are experiencing a higher risk of violence in the workplace. In fact, according to estimates reported by the Bureau of Labor Statistics (BLS), nonfatal assaults on hospital workers happened at a rate of 8.3 assaults per 10,000 workers. This was much higher than the rate in the general sector, which was two per every

The War on Doctors

10,000 workers for private-sector industries. Additionally, violence occurred during times of higher activity and interaction with the patients, such as during transport, mealtimes and during visiting hours. Some assaults take place because services are denied, or when restrictions are set on the patient, such as limiting eating, drinking, or tobacco use. Violence can range from offensive and threatening speech to murder. Workplace violence is specifically defined as violent acts directed to workers on duty. In other workplaces, such as convenience stores or taxicabs, robbery is more often the motive. In the hospital, violence usually comes from patients or their families and is often the result of frustration. Those who are in the most direct contact with patients, such as nurses, seem to be at the highest risk. The most common places for the violence to occur are on the psychiatry wards, in the emergency or waiting rooms and on the geriatric units.[1] Angry patients are indeed at war with doctors and other healthcare workers. This anger can often escalate into violence. We need to quash this war and protect our healthcare workers.

In *Psychiatric Times,* the statistics for healthcare workers in psychiatric settings is even more dismal. The rate of nonfatal crimes committed against psychiatrists was 66.2 per thousand. Of psychiatrists who were surveyed, 40% admitted being assaulted at some point in their careers. An example presented is this article is quite chilling: "At age 53, Wayne S. Fenton, MD, was a nationally recognized expert on the treatment of schizophrenia. He was an associate director at the NIMH. In addition, he maintained a private practice and treated patients with severe mental illness on weekday evenings and on weekends. Dr. Fenton was totally devoted to his patients.

On Saturday, September 2, 2006 (Labor Day Weekend) Dr. Fenton saw Vitali Davydov, aged 19, in consultation for treatment of severe psychosis. The father was present. On conclusion of the consultation, an appointment for treatment was made for later in the week. On Sunday, September 3, the patient's father called Dr. Fenton, pleading with him to see his son immediately. The son was agitated and angry about taking medications. At 4 pm, Dr. Fenton saw the patient in a small, private office behind a locked door. The father left to run an errand.

Dr. Fenton encouraged the patient to take an intramuscular long-acting antipsychotic. Upon the father's return, he found his son wandering about with blood on his hands. Dr. Fenton was discovered beaten to death." [2]

Angry patients are at war with doctors. Most patients, however, are appreciative of our efforts. However, just the few that lash out can lead to burnout and, in extreme cases, even homicide. While treating patients, our focus should be fully on the patient in front of us. It strains the relationship to deal with angry outbursts. Sure, patients are frustrated and need to let off steam. This is not what I am talking about here. We all understand that people come with emotions. I am talking about when it turns offensive or even violent. Often this anger is often against entities in the system but it is heaped on us, as we are the only players standing face-to-face with our patients. It is okay to express your anger or frustration. Just keep in mind, the doctor treating you is probably just as frustrated by the system. You may be angered by one test that has been denied, but the doctor bears the weight of many others. This war of angry patients wears us out and it shouldn't be that way. Let's all focus our attention on the source of our frustrations and try to effect change. Isn't it time to end this war and become a team again? Isn't it time we stand hand in hand with our patients and demand better care from the system? Isn't it time we refuse to keep being crushed under the out-of-control beast of a healthcare system?

1- http://www.cdc.gov/niosh/docs/2002-101/
2- http://www.psychiatrictimes.com/patient-violence-against-health-care-professionals

Chapter 6 TV Character Doctors

Standing in the passport line with my son, thoughts of *Grey's Anatomy* characters raced across my mind. I just noticed that I had a splotch of meatball sauce on the front of my shirt. As far as I could recall, no TV doctor walked around with food stains on their clothes because they had only five minutes to eat dinner. In fact, I tried to remember if I even remembered to comb my hair in the morning. Doctor characters on screen always appear so much more sophisticated. I think patients expect the same from real doctors.

Then there is Dr. House. I watch his show and am amazed at the diseases he diagnoses. It is just unbelievable. I mean really unbelievable—really, really unbelievable. Yet patients come and expect me to do what he does. They ask me about something they saw on Dr. House. I point out that I will not do what he does simply because he does not exist. He is a made-up, fictional character and his patients are not real either. To be fair, he came up with many more incorrect diagnoses than right ones. He was ornery as well.

Many patients have a hard time separating fact and fiction in these medical shows. It puts much more pressure on us and with it the expectation for perfection. This is a very unrealistic perfection. Doctors are human and we have lives outside of work just like everyone else. We go to our kids' soccer and basketball games, we go to PTA meetings, the gym, the beach, the grocery store, we shop, we pump our own gas, we celebrate holidays and attend family functions.

Patients don't always understand this. When I drive, I do not answer my phone. It is illegal, as simple as that. The police in New Jersey don't care if you are a doctor. If they see you with a cell phone out, you will be ticketed. After hours, the office phone line is transferred to one of our cell phones. On this particular day, I was on a mission to pick up school supplies for my daughter. My target destination was 10 minutes away. A patient literally called me every single minute for

15 minutes. I usually reply to messages in a very timely manner. She did not leave one. I answered when I arrived at my destination and she gave me an earful as I walked the aisles at Sam's Club of how she had been calling and getting no answer. I explained my policy about driving and answering messages. Apparently, this was unacceptable. It was 8 PM and she needed a refill of her medication right NOW. I explained I was not in the office and if she could ask the pharmacy to call me, I would give it to them right away over the phone. This too was not appropriate and I was supposed to be the one to look up the number and call. Of course, it would have been much easier if she had called during office hours. But many patients expect us to do their will whenever they need. This battle is wearing on many doctors, leading to burn out. We need mutual respect.

I was grocery shopping one day and I encountered a patient. Has anyone ever seen a TV doctor grocery shopping? The patient said that she was surprised that I shopped for my own groceries. I wondered who on earth would do it for me and who I could possibly trust enough to remember my secret stash of Peanut M&Ms. Yes, doctors do chores like everyone else. We wash dishes and mow the lawn. We don't all close our offices every Wednesday to play golf, as many assume. Many of these stereotypes are actually hurtful to many of us.

On TV, diseases are diagnosed in a 60-minute time period. That rarely happens in real life. Test results are slower to come back. Often, we must do multiple tests to arrive at the right diagnosis. Patients sometimes come in under the wrong assumption that they will get immediate answers to their concerns. Medicine only works that way on TV, not in real life.

I remember watching an episode of "ER" and the doctors in training diagnosed a patient with lung cancer based on a chest x-ray finding. My mind was saying no way. In real life, an abnormal chest x-ray would prompt further workups. The next step would most likely be a CT scan of the chest. It would take several days to weeks to make a diagnosis. Patients don't want to wait that long; they want an immediate diagnosis and I truly wish that were possible.

An article in *Time* discusses how fictional doctors on TV affect real patients. A team of researchers studied this question. They first did a survey of nurses and medical students and found that the vast majority of them felt that TV medicine bore little resemblance to real life medicine. They specifically examined the shows *House, MD* and *Grey's Anatomy*. In 50 episodes of these shows between the fall of 2005 and the spring of 2006, they identified 179 ethical dilemmas. Of these, 49 involved the issues of obtaining informed consent from patients or their loved ones. In 57% of the cases, the actors missed the mark completely. The researchers found 22 incidents where the TV characters veered deliberately from accepted practice. The incidents involved ignoring their own medical ethics and putting patients in harm's way needlessly. In one episode of *Grey's Anatomy*, one of the fictional doctors deliberately harms her patient (also her boyfriend) so that he would be moved up higher on the transplant list. The researchers found that only 5% of over 300 interactions between colleagues mirrored real life professional behavior. Of the doctor-patient interactions, only 1/3 bore any resemblance to reality. They found such a high incidence of sexual misconduct that they created a separate category for it and found much of it breeched professional standards.[1] So *House, MD* and *Grey's Anatomy* are clearly not the shows to watch if you wish to get a glimpse into the truth of the reality of medicine.

Another article in *The Atlantic* discusses how TV doctors shape perceptions. This article mentions the fact that several studies revealed that people who watched more medical shows were more likely to believe certain things about doctors and healthcare. Cultivation theory suggests that people cannot readily detect the difference between reality and the things they see on TV. The theory basically says that the social reality they witness on TV shapes their attitudes toward social reality. It often happens in complicated and not so obvious ways. In 2005, the CDC conducted a survey and found that the majority of primetime TV viewers admitted to learning something new about a disease or healthcare issue in the previous six months of viewing. Additionally, about 1/3 of them took some action about some health issue they learned about on TV. Though many shows now consult physicians, the shows are still filled with inconsistencies. These misconceptions can be outright dangerous, such as holding down a seizing patient and placing something in their mouth. Patients on TV tend to survive cardiac arrest much more commonly than they do in real life. People get the impression that CPR works much better than it actually does. These shows need to be filled with sensationalism to attract viewers: rare diseases, accidents, and natural disasters are a few examples. People get a skewed view of the problems in the healthcare world and important conditions such as diabetes get minimized. They can be seen as less important that the other more fantastic stories.[2]

These shows give people many false impressions—first, that common diseases are not so important, as they rarely receive any screen time. Rare diseases are solved in an hour episode and patients cured in the same period. In reality, rare disease patients can go years before they receive an accurate diagnosis. For many of them, there simply is no cure. People see the hyped-up heroics that doctors perform on TV and think doctors can do that in the real world. Sadly, that is not the case. When it comes to the point that a person needs CPR, the vast majority of them die. These shows also portray doctors in less ethical arrays. Many TV doctors do commit unethical behaviors. In real life, they would be reprimanded at the least, or even lose their medical licenses for such antics. The real world of medicine is not overflowing with sexual indiscretions. In real life, doctors are too tired and don't have any spare time.

A HoltzReport article examined some myths perpetuated by medical shows. One such myth is that doctors spend hours or days on one interesting patient. On *House, MD,* a whole team of healthcare workers devote their entire time to diagnosing one patient. This does not happen in real life. Doctors do not have time like this to devote

The War on Doctors

on a single patient. There is no team devoted to the care of one patient until he/she is diagnosed. This happens only on TV. Another myth is that "doctors do everything." However, in the real world, there are many other workers assisting in patient care: nurses, technicians and many more. *Grey's Anatomy,* for instance, shows the doctors putting their patients through the MRI scanner. In real life, technicians do this. The same goes for the doctors on *House, MD,* which depicts the doctors on the show processing their own lab samples. Again, in real life, skilled technicians perform these tasks. These shows are minimizing the work that the other members of the healthcare team perform. These other workers do work that is just as important and essential as the work doctors are doing. It is common on TV to see the fictional characters operating all the machinery. In real life, this work is done by technicians. Another myth is that it is common place to find doctors hooking up in storage closets or other places in the hospital. This only happens on TV because in reality, doctors would most likely be penalized for behaving inappropriately at work. As stated in the article, and bolstered by what I have witnessed in the real world, doctors remain focused on patient care while at work, and not their personal lives. On TV, most patients recover completely after a medical emergency. This is not the case as often in the real world. Many patients suffer long-term complications and doctors treat many more common diseases, such as diabetes and hypertension, than the medical heroics that are played out in the world of fiction. The last myth that this article examines is the one that tells us that TV viewers know what they are watching is fiction so it does not have to be accurate. The truth, however, is that these fictional shows do impact the public's perception. Many studies bore this out and showed that when certain diseases were discussed, there was a spike in public attention to them.[3]

Are these myths really harmful? I believe that they are for several reasons. One of the most important is that patients receive inaccurate medical information. I remember someone telling me, after watching *ER,* they could easily tell which patients needed a Z-pack. This was someone with no medical background. Based on watching these shows, patients may neglect to go for appropriate medical care or demand care that is unnecessary. People also see heroic saves from horrible diseases. While this does happen in real life, the assumption that this is the norm can be devastating when the opposite happens. People need to be aware that medical emergencies, particularly CPR, can often result in death. While these shows tend to show doctors in heroic fashion, it is important to keep in mind that all people working in the healthcare system play an essential role. I see it happen where a patient is rude to my staff and nice to me. I need my staff. I cannot practice medicine without them. I make it known to these patients that the office staff is not there to be abused. Fictional TV should do a better job reflecting the importance of everyone working in healthcare. These myths create a false scenario that doctors need to battle every day. We are at war with fictional medicine and medical characters as we strive to address concerns and save lives on the real world stage.

I am a doctor but don't play one on TV. No, I cannot diagnose rare diseases in one-hour increments. Nor can I fly into burning buildings and save all the inhabitants. I am a real doctor and I practice evidence-based medicine. I care about my patients. In my free time, I do not have exciting adventures. I do have kids, mow the lawn, do the grocery shopping and I even clean windows. Doctors are real people, just like everyone else. TV doctors are fiction and can never do what a real doctor is capable of doing. They may earn all the money, but I can make a real difference in the lives of my patients. It is fun to watch these shows. I do and provide my own commentary in the background, but it is important to remember the difference. When patients fall under the false expectations of these shows, it is another war we fight. In the end, we will win because we care more.

1- http://content.time.com/time/health/article/0,8599,1978591,00.html

The War on Doctors

2- http://www.theatlantic.com/health/archive/2014/08/healthcare-in-the-time-of-greys-anatomy/379087/

3- http://holtzreport.com/housemd/As_Seen_on_TV_Kirkwood%20Eagle-Tribune_20070305_HR.htm

Chapter 7 Celebrity Real Doctors and the Damage They Cause

Most doctors possess a special dislike for Dr. Oz. In fact, many think he should resign. It is not that he is a bad doctor; in fact, those who witnessed him perform surgery think that he is a very good one. However, it is his promotions of quackery that most of us object to. We all saw the news that he was called before Congressional hearings to defend his actions for promoting a weight loss drug that doesn't work. How many patients were scammed on that one? On his television show, he fields medical questions from his viewing audience and is held as a medical expert.

Yet the advice he gives is based on his own cult beliefs, and maybe the network's desire for higher rankings. He discounts science and real medicine. Why is this wrong? Many people embrace alternative medicine. But real medicine is a science as well as an art. Science has been proven in clinical trials to be effective and repetitive. In medicine, certain safety standards also are required to be met. Dr. Oz espouses his own special brand of "medicine," one he invented himself. There were no clinical trials nor was it proven effective, safe, or repetitive. Doctors like to refer to this type of medicine as "snake oil" medicine. Basically, it is anything that could be sold to make a profit if a person is so gullible as to fall for the false claims of its "magic"—i.e., a scam.

Seemingly, there exists a large enough population willing to be scammed to allow him to be successful, and this can lead to very real harm. While some people think that doctors just don't want any talk of alternative medicine, this is simply not true. We don't want people harmed.

Recently, the news carried the story of how several of his critics asked for his resignation from Columbia University. He responded on his show but his response was rather lackluster, addressing only one aspect of the criticism. He largely ignored many other doctors' questions.

The War on Doctors

Dr. Oz responded on his show to his "critics", the 10 doctors who petitioned Columbia Medical School for his resignation. He failed to respond, however, to many other doctor critics calling for his resignation. In fact, a poll conducted on SERMO (the largest social network exclusive to physicians) revealed that over 1500 doctors polled felt that he should resign from his position at Columbia University.

Throughout the years, Dr. Oz promoted many scientifically questionable methods. One of these, a weight loss product that he sold for profit, caused him to appear before a Congressional hearing to defend his behavior. He no longer deals in these specific products because they have not proven effective. Yet all those who purchased these products under the false assumption that they work were ripped off with no hope of recovering their lost dollars. They were fooled by someone who was supposed to be a trusted medical expert--basically, they were scammed.

After responding to his "critics," he stated that his show is not a "medical show." Yet, on his show, he dresses as a doctor and fields medical questions. The audience is under the assumption that they are addressing questions to a physician. So what would one call his show if not a medical show?

Dr. Oz has promoted the belief in communicating with deceased loved ones as a health benefit. He had a psychic medium appear on his show. He believes there are medical benefits to it, including lowering stress. Clearly, there are no clinical studies to back up his claims here.

Dr. Oz holds many such beliefs that are contrary to established medicine that he discusses on the show. Viewers have no way of knowing what is real medicine and what his is own cult medicine. They are likely to become victims of this pseudoscience without more expert information.

This false information is actually harmful in many ways:

- A person with a real medical problem may defer seeing a real medical doctor and getting real medical attention.
- A person may reject the best treatments based on false statements Dr. Oz has promoted on his show.

- A person is gullible in spending their hard-earned money on products that have no scientific basis. They are likely to become victims of being scammed.
- Wrong information can lead to wrong decisions.
- Dr. Oz is creating a show for viewership, not because he actually cares about the health of the viewers. The more sensational the better, whether it works or not. In contrast, real doctors care about the outcomes of their patients.
- Dr. Oz bears no liability in information he gives on his show. He can say whatever he wants with no repercussions. If a person is harmed, there is nothing that can be done.

Doctors spent many years studying and training to learn the science of medicine. We took an oath to do the best for our patients. We cannot throw all we learned out the window and make up our own "science" for the sake of making ourselves popular. This is simply unethical. As for celebrity doctors, they should be held to a higher standard because they have a larger audience. When a person places their trust in us as a physician, we need to honor that trust and provide the best medical information we know. If we forget how to do that, then perhaps it is best that Dr. Oz resign. Do we want celebrity doctors who invent their own science? Or do we want those who promote real medicine?

One patient recently was diagnosed with breast cancer. She saw something on a show of Dr. Oz that led her to believe that she wanted to forego traditional medicine. She asked me my advice. I asked her why she wanted to die. I then explained the evidence in regard to the treatment of breast cancer and that she was indeed diagnosed early enough and had a great prognosis. I spent over an hour with her trying to convince her not to go the way of Oz because that was a sure death sentence for her. She was 34 with two little kids and I kept picturing their sweet faces before me. I really wonder if Dr. Oz would have cared about her like that as much as his ratings. The advice he gives, like other celebrity doctors who chose to forego science and promote their own reality, wages war on doctors on the frontlines daily. Most of us wish they would go back to being real doctors and not just shooting for the stars. Peoples' lives are at stake. I am happy to say that my patient finally decided to embrace evidence-based medication and is doing well.

The War on Doctors

Recently, the BMJ (British Medical Journal) explored the truth of the recommendations offered by Dr. Oz on his show. To physicians, it was hardly surprising, as we have had the task of fighting off these false beliefs for some time now. The *BMJ* found that approximately 50% of his recommendations were baseless or outright wrong. What is more concerning is that 15% of the advice he gives is contradicted by medical evidence. For this study, researchers from Canada analyzed health claims they randomly selected from 40 episodes of *Dr. Oz* and *The Doctors.* They identified over 900 recommendations made on both of these shows. They then randomly selected 80 recommendations from each show and analyzed each based on medical evidence. The results specifically from the *Dr. Oz* show revealed that only 46% of his recommendations could be supported with evidence. Additionally, 15% were outright contraindicated by the medical evidence and 39% did not have any evidence either way. The recommendations that were made provided very little context to the viewers, meaning they would be acting without full knowledge of the risks and benefits for their particular situation.[1] So when your doctor tells you not to listen to the advice from Dr. Oz, we are not saying that just because we do not like the man. We are following evidence-based medicine. We are practicing the real science and not the made for TV pseudoscience. Is Dr. Oz standing there on the screen because he cares if you, the viewer, achieve good health? No, he is doing it to make money, just like the supplements he sells.

Today, a patient came in to request a serum iodine level because she saw it on a "medical TV show." She told me that she had every single symptom they listed and she KNEW she had iodine deficiency. I explained that anyone living in the US would not be iodine deficient because salt here is fortified with it. She insisted that she does not add salt on to her food just to further her theory. I explained that most food is cooked with some salt. I have never, in fact, ordered an iodine level on anyone before because it is not needed. But this TV celebrity doctor said it was so, and if he is on TV, he must be right.

Dr. Sears is a famous pediatrician and an author of many books. It is a shame that he doesn't stand for all pediatricians because children are in need of strong advocates these days. In an article in *Science-Based Medicine,* it is suggested that Dr. Sears capitalizes on the fear of parents and going against the establishment. One of these fears that he seems to profit greatly off of is fear of vaccines. He seems to write what parents want to hear, rather than speaking up for evidence-based medicine. He supports not vaccinating kids and even developing individualized immunization schedules. He is branding himself as the only true expert who knows how to safely give vaccines. He spreads untruths, myths, and fear-mongering to already concerned parents. He has denounced the guidelines of the American Academy of Pediatrics and the CDC and states that his vaccination schedule is better and safer. Yet he has no evidence. There have been no studies to examine his claims. He continues to sell books with these untruths. He downplays the true seriousness of the diseases these vaccines are preventing. He suggests that vaccinating against diphtheria is no longer needed in the US because it no longer is prevalent. According to the author of this article, Dr. Sears demonstrates a poor understanding of epidemiology and public health. The author then proceeds to dispel the myths one by one and provide sound scientific reasoning, which is lacking in Dr. Sears' made up immunization schedule.[2]

Dr. Sears is dangerous. While many see him as a well-known pediatrician, he is promulgating dangerous myths. Children still die from vaccine-preventable diseases. Just recently, a child in Europe died from diphtheria. His parents were opposed to vaccinating. As physicians, we need to be the experts. However, that does not give us the right to make up our own brand of medicine or science. There are clinical studies that need to be cited. We need to practice evidence-based medicine. The efficacy and safety of vaccines has been well established for decades. When a well-known doctor debunks that science, he is putting lives in jeopardy, in this case the lives of infants and young children. Every day, I promote vaccines to my patients. However, they will sometimes quote Dr. Sears to me. No, I am not going to read any of his books. He is just downright wrong. This is a very real war doctors carry out with celebrity doctors. As medical experts, we need to speak out and give sound science to the public, not boost book sales.

Another of these celebrity doctors to review is Dr. Drew Pinsky, commonly known as Dr. Drew. He is a practicing physician who is board certified in internal medicine and addiction medicine. He is also the host of the reality show *Celebrity Rehab with Dr. Drew.* On the show, celebrities with addiction receive treatment from other celebrities on TV. Without examining anything else, I think this can be seen as obviously exploitive of real serious problems. What is the benefit for Dr. Drew to do it live on TV? Does anyone honestly feel that this is in the best interests of those suffering addiction? Or is it about the money?

An article in *The Atlantic* explores how Dr. Drew sold out to the pharmaceutical companies. It discusses his other media ventures: *Loveline,* a radio show about sexual health and a nightly program for HLN. The pharmaceutical company Glaxo-Smith Kline (GSK) has been fined in the amount of $3 billion. They were found guilty of a wide range of violations, from illegal marketing to misreporting drug prices. Dr. Drew was not found guilty of any crime, but he was an enabler in these activities. He deceived his audiences as part of a program for GSK through town meetings, writings, and media appearances. "Aware that Wellbutrin's main competition, the class of drugs known as SSRIs, came with the unfortunate risk of lowering libido, GSK's sales department developed an ingenious plan to use Dr. Pinsky as the face of a public education campaign getting the word out about these side effects and other effective antidepressants that do not disrupt sexual desire and function," as GSK's website said. Other antidepressants then available that didn't seem to depress sex drive included Serzone, which is now off the market, and Remeron. But both had other complicating factors that made Wellbutrin the better choice in such situations. He hasn't issued any apology but stated it was based on his own clinical experience. It is important to keep in mind that Dr. Drew was speaking to the general public who trusted him as a source of medical information. So while he was broadcasting wrong information favoring GSK's product, he also failed to mention that he was speaking on behalf of them,[3] a clear violation of ethics in healthcare. All speakers must disclose their conflicts of interest. Being a celebrity does not exempt him from that.

Then there is the issue of one of his former celebrity addicts, Mindy McCready, who had been a patient on his show. She ended up committing suicide. In fact, she was the fifth former cast member to die.[4] One has to wonder if she and the others would have met the same fate if they received treatment out of the spotlight. In fact, psychotherapy is a very important component of treating addiction. In order to achieve success with it, there needs to be a very strong therapeutic relationship between the patient and the doctor. How is this even possible to attempt on live TV? Many would find this ethically reprehensible. But there is money to be made here. As the doctor in this relationship, Dr. Drew has a higher ethical responsibility to assure patients receive appropriate care but instead, he exploits their suffering for monetary gain on reality TV.

Another celebrity doctor that has thrown away medical integrity for personal gain is Dr. Joseph Mercola. Dr. Mercola is an osteopathic physician who advertises himself as an alternative medicine proponent. He sells a variety of supplements and medical devices through his website, which is one of the most trafficked sites in healthcare.

Many of the products that Dr. Mercola sells bear his own name. The problem is that many of these products don't work, yet he claimed they did. In 2005, the FDA ordered him to stop making false claims. He received a second warning letter from the FDA in 2006 after they investigated some of the labels on his products. Some of them proposed to reduce the risk of cancer. In 2011, the FDA again ordered him to stop making false claims, this time regarding the use of thermography. He claimed on his site that this device could detect various diseases, even cancer. He intended to fight this but apparently stopped using thermography in his practice.[5]

Science-Based Medicine published an article on reasons to completely ignore Dr. Mercola. This article pretty much labels Mercola.com "a horrible chimera of tabloid journalism, late-night infomercials, and amateur pre-scientific medicine." Dr. Mercola, despite the vast body of evidence supporting vaccinations, makes several false claims of why they are not needed. He recommended not getting the swine flu vaccine because it was not a deadly disease, yet 36,000 people died from it. He accuses public health officials of being negligent in failing to inform the public on how to boost their immunity against influenza. He makes the claim that Amish children, who are not vaccinated, do not get afflicted with autism, suggesting that is the cause. He is wrong on all accounts. Vaccines have clearly been shown not to be the cause of autism, Amish people do vaccinate their kids, and they do have kids who suffer from

The War on Doctors

Autism. He makes many other false vaccine claims.[6] His site is full of false claims about many other things as well. He has a host of products with no proven benefit that he is profiting from.

Is it wrong for doctors to be celebrities? Absolutely not! But being in the spotlight, they need to realize that the general public looks to them as trusted medical experts. They should be held to a high standard, as their advice is reaching literally millions of minds. Does it bother me when a patient comes in believing a fallacy that they learned from Dr. Oz? It sure does. I am usually able to convince them of the evidence because they know me and we have developed a relationship of mutual trust. However, the issue that concerns me is that so many people are being led astray by celebrities touting false claims. Not only are they being scammed and wasting their hard-earned money by purchasing products with no proven benefit, but they are being put in harm's way. Legally, I am held to following the standard of medical care. What this means is that I am expected to, and will be held legally responsible for, practicing medicine in the same way as my peers in my specialty practice. If I stray from this standard, I can be held liable for any harm caused by doing so. Doctors are scientists. There are whole bodies of scientific research showing the evidence of what is safe and effective. I cannot ignore these truths and create my own science. Yet that is what many of these celebrity doctors are doing. They are selling products that do not work, making false claims about things that are proven and denouncing life-saving procedures such as vaccinations. They don't do this because they discovered evidence supporting their claims. The reason that they do this is because it is popular and they are trying to try up their ratings. The more traffic they generate, the more products they sell, the more media opportunities they receive and they earn more money. It is as simple as that.

As you watch the TV doctor, keep in mind that they do not know you or care about you. You are just a viewer to them and a potential customer. They hold no incentive to solve your medical problems. They are at war with real doctors trying to do the best for our patients using real evidence-based medicine. Real doctors do care about our patients. If you don't feel that way with your personal doctor, find one who will make you feel that way. TV doctors are held in very high esteem despite the fact that they sold their integrity to make profits. It doesn't matter how famous they are or that it is "just a TV show." We all took the Hippocratic Oath. We all vowed to do no harm. These doctors are doing very real harm by giving out false medical information. We need to call them to step up to the standard. We cannot allow them to continue practicing their own snake oil medicine on people. We need real doctors giving out real medical information. Patients deserve better and should demand more dedication to their health from the doctors on TV. Isn't it time we changed channels?

1- https://www.advisory.com/daily-briefing/2014/12/19/bmj-about-50-of-dr-ozs-recommendations-are-baseless-or-wrong
2- https://www.sciencebasedmedicine.org/cashing-in-on-fear-the-danger-of-dr-sears/
3- http://www.theatlantic.com/health/archive/2012/07/how-dr-drew-sold-his-cred-to-big-pharma/259473/
4- http://www.goodtherapy.org/blog/topic-expert-round-up-dr-drew-dr-phil-rehab-TV-draw-ire-0312135
5- http://www.quackwatch.com/11Ind/mercola.html
6- https://www.sciencebasedmedicine.org/9-reasons-to-completely-ignore-joseph-mercola-and-natural-news/

8 Just Sue the Doctor

People think that if anything goes wrong with their health, that they will just sue their doctor. Why not? The doctor has malpractice insurance. It must be some kind of "share the wealth" thinking. But what they don't realize is how destructive a lawsuit can be. First, it is undue stress and disrupts the life and time of the doctors for an extended period of time. Who can practice good medicine with lawyers circling around? If the suit is lost, the doctor is reported in something called the National Practitioner's Data Bank (NPDB). No doctor wants to be listed there. It is like a doctor's death sentence. Once listed there, a doctor gets a black mark and finds it harder to get a job, hospital privileges, liability insurance, and much more. So no, never just sue the doctor because your C-section scar, which you signed the consent form for and were made aware of all the complications before it was done, didn't heal up in two days.

Therefore, the threat to sue the doctor is a battle, always waging war on us. Patients use this threat frequently. I recently saw a new patient in her 30s who demanded a prescription for 100 tablets of Oxycodone. Well, first, I never prescribed 100 tablets of that medication in my life. Second, I never prescribe controlled substances to a patient on a first visit. All too often, patients lie, especially when they are trying to score their medication of the day. Plus, New Jersey now has a controlled substance reporting system and doctors can look up all the prescriptions for these types of medications that were filled. And look her up I did. She had 21 pages of prescriptions filled from five different doctors. I explained this to her and she said that someone else must have been using her identity. I offered to call the police to report this very serious identity theft. At that point, she became aggressive and told me that if I did not give her the prescription and she went into withdrawal, she would sue me. I explained it would actually be the other doctors who would be liable as they were the ones who got her addicted and I offered her a referral to a rehab program. Needless to say, she stormed out empty-handed. But, this threat of lawsuit is a nasty one and doctors should not be threatened needlessly like this.

But the real war is more with the lawyers than the patients. How many times have you been watching television when an advertisement just pops up instructing you to call this lawyer if you were harmed by medication xyz? Many of these are for medications that are still commonly prescribed and effective. There is no scientific proof that they cause harm. But if lawyers are taking cases to litigate, it must be a dangerous drug, right? Pharmaceutical companies make big profits so they make good targets for lawsuits. These lawyers are basically on a fishing expedition that will land them the big case. But this is truthfully quite harmful because it eliminates some good choices of medications our patients can use because they are now afraid of it.

In another conversation that I overheard (no, I do not eavesdrop, people just have loud voices sometimes), one woman was telling another that if the surgery did not go well, she could just sue the doctor. The other woman said that she liked her doctor and wouldn't think of doing that. But the other woman told her that it would just come from the malpractice insurance and no harm would come to her beloved physician.

We live in a lawsuit-friendly society. Everyone looks to cast blame when something goes wrong. Have you ever been in an automobile accident? Then you know that the police report is public record and soon followed by an onslaught of letters from lawyers trying to represent you in filing a claim for your injuries. Where there is a bad outcome, people are looking for someone to blame. Often, the finger is pointed at the doctor and the medical team. The realization that every procedure has the possibility of a bad outcome despite the best possible care goes unrecognized. This is despite the fact that patients sign consent forms explaining all the risks of a given procedure and confirming that they are aware of these possible bad outcomes. They just never believe that it can happen to them. Since it is expected in only a small percentage of cases, surely something must have been done wrong. But most often, this is not the case.

The War on Doctors

According to the AMA, more than 61% of doctors over the age of 55 have been sued at least once. Approximately 10-20% of cases occur because of a missed diagnosis. The malpractice litigation hits some specialties harder than others. For example, general surgeons and OB/GYN doctors tend to be sued the most. Almost 70% of doctors in these specialties have been sued at least once and 50% have been sued 2 or more times. The least likely to be sued are pediatricians and psychiatrists. While there are a large number of suits, few of these result in any payments and doctors most often win the cases when they go to court. Most cases never make it to the courtroom but are settled prior to going to trial. In 2012, payouts from lost malpractice cases resulted in payouts of $3.6 billion.[1]

It is not just the direct effect of litigation that drives up healthcare costs. A recent Gallop poll showed that approximately 1 out of every 4 healthcare dollars goes into defensive medicine. An independent healthcare economics firm, BioScience Valuation, estimates the annual cost of defensive medicine exceeds $480 billion. RAND Corporation reported that 3 states adapted tort reform hoping to show a reduction in healthcare spending that ERs spend toward defensive medication. They failed to show any difference.[2]

Malpractice suits are damaging in many ways, not just to a physician's reputation. It causes untold stress upon the physician being sued and contributes to burnout. The less burnout that is present, the better a doctor will be. These suits take countless hours and take time away from face-to-face patient care. It also harms the doctor-patient relationship, not just with the patient filing the lawsuit. When a doctor is sued for unreasonable cause, they begin to distrust their patients. The doctor-patient relationship is one based on trust, going both ways. The more the trust, the stronger the relationship will be.

I know many OB/GYN doctors have stopped delivering babies because they are no longer able to afford their malpractice premium payments. The risk of being sued for delivering a baby with problems has gotten to be too costly for many doctors. This is harmful because we are decreasing our pool of available OB/GYN doctors. While everyone is saddened when a baby has complications, there is often no way to prevent them from happening. Yet this represents a big area of liability. I know of one OB/GYN who lost everything after being sued. At the time the suit was filed, her malpractice carrier filed for bankruptcy. This essentially left her uninsured. She lost her home and most of her savings in this suit. She was not even the primary obstetrician in the delivery of this baby. She was just on-call and covering for another physician. The delivery was uneventful, yet the baby was born with cerebral palsy. As physicians, we know that not all cases of CP result from birth trauma. Sometimes, despite the best medical care, babies are born with this disease and there is no way to prevent it. Yet doctors are often found liable for babies born with CP, whether they are at fault or not. She no longer delivers babies although she is a fine doctor.

No doctor should be threatened for going against their better judgment. We should not feel pressured to practice medicine under the threat of litigation. For one thing, it drives up healthcare costs for unnecessary care. It is just bad medicine and not in the best interests of our patients. Yet these types of stories are happening frequently all across the country. Patients need protection from malpractice and medical negligence but it must be a fair process. It has strayed far from its intended course. Doctors can be sued for any reason without any evidence of wrongdoing. Jury decisions are often decided by emotional factors and not medical facts. While everyone is trying to cure the problem of the uninsured and the burden they place on our healthcare system, there will be no healthcare reform without tort reform.

How can we achieve relevant tort reform in the healthcare system?

- One thing that can be considered is a system of arbitration rather

  than taking these cases through the judicial system.

- We need to eliminate frivolous lawsuits. These drive up liability

  costs and serve no useful purpose.

The War on Doctors

- The loser in a malpractice case should pay the litigation costs. This is a way to ensure that only serious cases are brought to trial.

- Verdicts in malpractice cases should be decided by a jury of peers, meaning medical professionals, not the general public. This would help ensure that outcomes are determined by medical facts and not emotion.

- There should be financial caps on awards.

Our litigious society is contributing to the high healthcare costs in the US. One quarter of healthcare dollars has been estimated to go toward the practice of defensive medicine. Many studies are ordered out of fear of liability. When we see that the majority of lawsuits are filed because of missed diagnoses, it is easy to understand this. Malpractice premiums have gone through the roof and many doctors are struggling to pay them. If this upward trend continues, some doctors may soon stop performing high-risk procedures. We are already seeing this in the field of OB/GYN where many doctors have stopped delivering babies because of the malpractice risk. We are losing many highly skilled doctors because of this. Tort reform needs to be addressed if we truly want healthcare reform. It is another symptom of our broken healthcare system. Doctors should be able to practice good medicine without the threat of lawsuit always hanging over their heads. Sure, patients need remedy if they have been faulted. But the medical malpractice system has overstepped its bounds. Do we want doctors providing the best medical treatments for our patients because we care about them? Or would we rather have doctors who practice to avoid litigation?

Lawyers are at war with doctors. They feel that we are a potential source of income for them. They try to make up cases. They advertise against us. They seek patients who take certain medications to start class action suits where the payouts are huge. They possess no real interest in helping the patient get justice but are rather seeking their own fame and monetary gain. There is a target on the backs of doctors from the legal system. It has forced us to practice defensive medicine, which is medicine practiced to avoid being sued. This drives up the costs of healthcare spending. But as long as there are lawyers out there looking at doctors through their crosshairs, we must continue doing this. Patients should receive compensation when they were injured in the medical system. But lawyers should stop inventing victims where there are none. Courts should step up and throw out cases without merit in a better fashion than they have been doing. This drives up court and legal costs as well. This war is more like open hunting season on healthcare specialists. We need to rein it in.

1- http://www.physicianspractice.com/blog/ten-notable-physician-related-malpractice-statistics

2- http://www.forbes.com/sites/theapothecary/2014/11/05/dont-reform-the-malpractice-system-to-reduce-healthcare-costs-eliminate-it/2/

Chapter 9 Our War with Each Other

Doctors like to joke that if you have a meeting with five doctors, you will get 10 different opinions. Over the last several years, the professional divide among doctors has widened. There exist doctors in all kinds of practice settings, from private practice business owners to employed doctors to those just putting in a few hours to keep busy past retirement. Each setting carries its own kind of stress and discord. Doctors in private practice struggle to keep their doors open with rising overhead costs and stagnant or decreasing reimbursements. Those in employed positions are often in opposition to the administrators in charge. They feel that their daily workloads are not understood by those in charge and feel pressure to comply with situations that they don't necessarily agree with. It's no wonder doctors disagree on many things.

If that is not enough, doctors feel that their medical organizations are at war with them. The largest one, the American Medical Association or AMA, lost favor among a great number of physicians. Yet for the most part, the public sees the AMA as the voice of physicians. The doctors of the AMA and those outside the organization are at great odds with each other. Approximately 80% of doctors in the US do not belong to the AMA. It is clear that the majority of doctors are being overridden by the minority. Many doctors believe that this must change.

The American Medical Association is all over the media as representing the voice of doctors. Even politicians cite AMA statistics in driving healthcare policy. But the fact is, physicians disagree. We do not believe the AMA represents us in anything, and doctors left their memberships in large numbers. In fact, it is estimated that only 15-18% of doctors in the US are paying members of the AMA. In one study conducted by Jackson and Coker, only 11% of physicians who responded believe the AMA stands for the views of doctors. Where did the AMA go astray on the path of representing physicians? Perhaps the biggest example of how doctors lost their trust in the AMA is the way they are funded. With less than 20% of US doctors paying membership dues, it is apparent they secure funding from other sources. One of their biggest streams of revenue is their profits from selling billing coding, insurance, and other products. Most doctors disagree with the CPT billing transformation. Yet the AMA continues to profit hugely from selling these products despite our protests. Clearly, doctors' opinions have been shoved underfoot in their quest to drive profits. The AMA is very ineffective at lobbying. One of the greatest examples can be seen in the SGR debacle playing out over decades. They were unable to change or influence any policy change. In fact, doctors feel that they sided with the politicians more often than with practicing doctors. Again, we were not represented by the AMA here. Doctors feel abused by insurance company policies. Reimbursements have been shrinking and often we are fighting to get paid for services we have provided. Here too, the AMA has offered little help. This is perhaps one of the biggest factors driving doctors out of private practice. Yet they stand mute on slowing down the flow of doctors out of their own practices. Mandates coming out of the government are intruding into the practice of medicine. The AMA does not hear doctors' concerns here but rather stands for itself. They throw their weight behind the politicians they chose rather than the mass of physicians. We feel the AMA would sell us out in a heartbeat.

The media often quotes the AMA as being the voice of doctors. Yet less than 20% of physicians in our country are even members. When doctors see these things in the media, it further tears down our trust because we have not been asked where we stand on the issues, while they are speaking up that they are representing us. No, they are not and the media and general public need to learn that the AMA no longer represents the majority of doctors in the US. Perhaps it is time for them to investigate what they have done to drive doctors away. The healthcare landscape in the US is rapidly evolving. Many changes have appeared that are harmful to our profession and patients alike. Doctors have no organization that truly represents what we are going through and none to drive truly beneficial reform. While doctors burn out from lack of guidance and enforced compliance with unreasonable mandates and guidelines driving insurance company profits, the AMA speaks out while

The War on Doctors

ignoring our plight and our voices. The AMA is not the voice of doctors and it is time that people stop recognizing them as anything other than a political organization shaping reforms and selling products off the backs of doctors for their own agendas and profits. Does anyone know an organization that is willing to stand up and be the real voice of doctors and help mold real healthcare reform?

In fact, the majority of doctors feel that most of our medical organizations do not represent doctors. More often than not, they are too seeped in politics to be effective change agents on behalf of doctors. While we need to be involved in politics to some degree to change healthcare policy, we need to retain our own voices. Doctors know what is best for patients in the exam room, more than politicians do. Many of our societies seem to be trying to get us to adapt to the agenda of their chosen political advocate. They are misrepresenting us in this fashion. Unless they truly step up to represent what doctors need, more and more doctors will be dropping their memberships.

It is not just that our societies fail to truly represent us; they often don't even listen to us. There is major controversy in the media lately regarding the maintenance of certification (MOC) program. The vast majority of doctors disagree with it and many are speaking out against it. Despite the fact that of doctors polled on SERMO, only 3% of them agreed with the MOC program, the leaders of the ABMS (American Board of Medical Specialties) continues to cling to their ways with fierce tenacity and continues to force us to comply. Is there any greater war among doctors than this?

While the medical boards have stated that complying with the MOC requirements is voluntary, this simply is not true. It is now necessary to complete the MOC requirements to be board-certified in your specialty. Most hospitals across the USA require doctors to be board-certified to maintain their staff privileges at the hospital, without which the doctor cannot treat patients inside the hospital. Additionally, in order to be on insurance panels, a physician must be board-certified and/or have hospital privileges in order to treat patients and earn a living. There is

71

simply no way out of having board certification, unless you have a cash-only outpatient practice.

Why do doctors not want to comply with MOC requirements?

1. The majority of doctors believe it is not relevant to the everyday practice of medicine. We feel we are forced to learn facts that are not used in clinical practice but are merely academic points. Therefore, the MOC is not really testing a physician's competency, as it claims. Rather, it is requiring physicians to memorize irrelevant medical minutiae.
2. It is costly. In order to maintain compliance with MOC, you have to pay the board. Some doctors have estimated over the course of a career, this could total more than $20,000 just to the board. Then there are the thousands of dollars for the study materials and the courses to attend to prepare for these requirements.
3. It is time consuming. The board claims it takes less than 20 hours per year to remain compliant. This simply is not true. Since it requires doctors to go back and memorize trivial facts that they do not need to practice quality medicine, they need to study, and this requires time. As the country's physician shortage grows, should doctors be taking time away from patients to study those things which they do not find beneficial?
4. There are no studies proving that the MOC improves patient care or clinical outcomes. As doctors, we are increasingly called to practice evidence-based medicine. Shouldn't the boards be held to the same standards?
5. Many doctors feel that the requirements are being developed by academic doctors and not those actively practicing medicine. Shouldn't the requirements to determine whether doctors are competent to practice medicine be devised by doctors who are actually practicing clinical medicine?
6. The boards claim that patients want these requirements and trust the board certification. No, my patients want me

to listen to their concerns and spend more time with them. They don't want me to be out of the office trying to prepare for the MOC when they are sick. Many of my patients do not know what board certification is. Many do. But the doctor-patient relationship is one based on trust that is built over time in a relationship. It is not forged by a certificate hanging on the exam room wall.

7. The leaders of the specialty medical boards are making exorbitant salaries, 3-4 times what a physician in clinical practice is making. Clearly, they have a financial conflict of interest in keeping the MOC going. Many doctors wonder how much of our MOC dollars are going into their pockets. Perhaps it is time for them to disclose their financial conflict of interest and make it transparent how much they are earning from this endeavor.

Some doctors are going so far as to say the medical boards are extorting doctors. We have no choice but to comply if we want to remain in practice. We have no say in setting the standards. No one listens to our opinions of how the MOC process can be made more relevant. Surely, such a process as this, that physicians are essentially forced into against our will, should not be making other people rich. Is this extortion or no? Clearly, the board needs to make some changes because the doctors' revolt is coming.

For many months, doctors cried out 'the ABIM is not listening to our concerns!' Most of us disagree with the forced MOC we need to comply with. Yet, the ABIM continues to turn deaf ears. In response to a *Newsweek* article by Kurt Eichenwald, they stated that the only doctors complaining are the ones active on social media. They claim doctors in the real world love MOC. This completely ignores the 23,000+ doctors who have signed a petition to abolish the MOC process. Why overlook these doctors' concerns? Perhaps the ABIM's financial bubble prevents them from hearing.

Information continues to leak out about the ABIM's financial irregularities. Why, for instance, do they possess a luxury condo that cost over one million dollars? A condo that was purchased from the money paid by the same doctors who oppose MOC yet are bound to meet requirements. Many articles exist decrying the financial constraints of the MOC process. Yet the ABIM executives persist in raking it in and ignoring members' feedback.

Many doctors believe that MOCs do not offer any real educational value. There is no evidence that shows that MOC provides any improved patient outcomes. It would seem intuitive that the ABIM would provide evidence of the validity of enforcing MOC on physicians in response to the *Newsweek* article. Rather, they cast blame on the author for not disclosing that his wife is an internist. The ABIM has very strict rules regarding disclosing conflicts of interest. This was not one of them but rather invented to attack this particular author.

The ABIM also cast blame on the author for not disclosing that his article was an opinion piece. The author published this as his weekly opinion column. It completely befuddles the mind why ABIM cast this accusation at the author rather than providing any support for the validity of MOC. Doctors reject the ABIM's claims that MOC improves clinical outcomes, especially as they failed to offer any reasonable evidence. As a doctor, when I prescribe a medication for a patient, I evaluate the evidence that it will work for the patient. Doctors step up to meet demands to practice evidence-based medicine daily. Why should the ABIM be held to different standards?
Doctors who questioned the ABIM were labeled "complainers" or the "usual suspects." Why would doctors be so easily dismissed when they were asking legitimate questions? Clearly, the monopoly of the ABIM allows them this luxury. They claim MOC is voluntary. However, this in reality is not true. If doctors remain uncertified by their specialty board, those doctors cannot have hospital privileges. Without hospital privileges, insurance companies disallow them from participating. In essence, our compliance is forced if we wish to continue practicing medicine. How can this be voluntary?

The revelation of the financial interests of the ABIM is appalling. Their profits remain in the tens of millions. Isn't this perhaps the biggest financial conflict of interest out there? While doctors pay the price under enslavement to the boards, they continue to generate huge profits for themselves. There is no obligation for them to provide evidence that they produce a beneficial service to doctors or patients alike. They extort physicians with no oversight. How is this not criminal?

I believe good always wins out over evil in the end. The ABIM erred when they silenced doctors and abused them for their own profits. They erred when not publishing evidence of why the MOC is necessary; they chose to attack a reporter writing an opinion piece and went after his wife. They succeeded in their corruption for a few years. But I predict their financial bubble will soon burst.

When most people think of doctors, there exists a certain stereotype of highly educated professionals with certain ethical standards. Sure, outliers exist in countless medical settings who give the rest of us bad names. Then there are those who not only manipulate the system for their own gain, but also abuse their fellow physicians for their own profit—the shady leaders of life-long learning.

No one would argue that doctors need to continue their education throughout their careers to stay abreast of the latest medical information and innovation. For years, we have been doing this by meeting required hours of CME (continuing medical education) to comply with our state medical licensing boards. Most doctors do not have any objection to this because it bears relevancy to our daily practices. In fact, we still do this although other requirements have been added on.

A few years ago, the ABMS (American Board of Medical Specialties, which oversees 24 approved medical specialty boards) stepped in. A new program was rolled out where doctors are now required to adhere to the MOC (Maintenance of Certification) program. The vast majority of doctors disagree with this process as it is costly, time consuming, and does not reflect medicine in the real world. In fact, of doctors polled on SERMO, the largest social media network exclusive to physicians, only 3% of doctors felt the MOC process worked well.

Over the last several months, there have been numerous articles and blog posts decrying doctors' disagreement with the medical boards and the MOC process. In fact, 23,000+ doctors signed a petition to the ABIM to end the MOC process. The ABIM persists in turning a deaf ear and defending themselves, although there is no evidence that the MOC process is actually an effective educational tool or improves clinical outcomes.

One may wonder why the ABIM fails to acknowledge members' concerns. But their finances slowly leaked out to the press. Their profits are in the tens of millions and their executives earn obscene salaries. Additionally, there is the question of that luxury condo that they claim as an investment. Many irregularities appear when looking through the ABIM's and the ABIM foundation's 990s. Interestingly, they filed an extension for their 2014 990 submissions.

The ABIM and all the medical specialty boards hold physicians hostage. We have no choice but to acquiesce to these requirements if we desire to keep practicing medicine. We are disallowed from treating patients at most hospitals or contracting with insurance companies if we are not board certified. Our careers are monopolized by the ABIM and other specialty boards without oversight. They possess the freedom to reap as much profit from us as they like without any accountability. The shady leaders of medical education abused us for the past few years. This is about to end because the whole truth is coming. Doctors will prevail and our voices will be heard.

The controversy regarding MOC (maintenance of certification) flourishes. However, there is not so much controversy as much as there is opposition. The ABIM continually ignores the doctors speaking out against the process. They label the dissident voices as complainers. They act as though we are wayward children who they need to educate for our own good because we are not capable of doing it ourselves. The simple fact is that only 3% of doctors polled on SERMO (the largest social network exclusive for physicians) agreed with the MOC process. So, with only 3% supporting their viewpoints, they call out the 97% as disruptive and unruly. Why? It is all about the money. Anyone following the news witnessed the corruption that leaked into the management of the ABIM. As if that weren't bad enough, a new low was whipped out by a former ABIM board member, Dr. Robert Wachter.

The War on Doctors

In his most recent blog article, he calls out the anti-MOC troops, as he calls the 97% who found some fault with the ABIM and MOC process. He calls us unhappy. Didn't know they were psychoanalyzing us as we write and tweet. Perhaps he thinks we should all start on Prozac? No, I am not unhappy. I, in fact, am a very happy person. I just call injustice when I see it.

The rest of his post tries to detail where he and the 3% are correct and the rest of the 97% wayward children strayed. He concludes his article comparing those who voice their opposition to the MOC process to the protesters of the Arab Spring. This is a foul and offensive comparison. My husband is Egyptian and most of his family and friends still live there. We know people who DIED standing up to a corrupt regime. Many that we know are still suffering in the crashed economy that resulted after the Arab Spring. The youth graduating college cannot find jobs and children cannot afford bread to eat. Some children cannot get an education because they are needed to work to support their families. Police officers were attacked and killed in the line of duty. Schools were closed for weeks at a time. Churches that were more than a thousand years old were destroyed and set on fire. People hid in their homes, afraid to step out in the streets for fear of their lives. Just earlier today (June 29, 2015), the former chief prosecutor, who tried and jailed many Muslim Brotherhood members, was assassinated in a car bomb in Cairo. There are expectations that the Brotherhood, in retaliation, will step up their fighting once again. But they do not do theirs by tweeting or writing blog posts. They use pipe bombs and knives. They throw innocent people from roofs of tall buildings. The country sits in uncertainty, as it has for the past several years.

Really, do we want to make this comparison of someone speaking up against something they see as unfair to people being killed? I find it offensive, not just to the Egyptian people but to dear friends who lost their lives in the Arab Spring. Should the atrocities that were committed during this revolution be so trivialized? What has civilization come to if someone's death is equated to a mere disagreement?

This is perhaps the biggest war between physicians at the moment. But there are others going on as well. This is preventing us from being effective change agents. If we really want to change the system, we need to come together and find our collective voice. With everything battling us these days, we should not be fighting amongst ourselves. We need to listen to each other. Isn't it time to end this war?

The War on Doctors

Chapter 10 Everyone Wants a Piece of Us

It was another boring sales lunch. Except that this sales rep didn't actually bring lunch but I was meeting him anyway. He was selling a hemoglobin analyzer. I would be able to bill the insurance company for the test and profit about...$1.80. His company would profit much more from the test strips that I would buy from him. When I pointed out that this was not even a break-even proposition, given that I would need my staff to do it and that it would not be done by itself, he pointed out that it would be a service to my patients and they wouldn't have to go to the lab. Except that we already drew blood in the office and sent it to the lab so his machine had no benefit to me. But he kept pushing and pushing. He left without a sale, and I was left without lunch and feeling used.

This is the trend I am seeing these days from salespeople and manufacturers. They try to give just a tiny profit to the doctors doing the work to get them interested, and they rake in the rest of the larger pot for themselves. Some days, I feel like the camel in the desert carrying everyone's goods on my back. Yet many of these devices are not even very helpful to us. They have been developed without input from doctors. We are just the target for their potential profits. It is another battle we face: attacks from greedy industry.

My LinkedIn in box is full of messages from healthcare start-ups asking me to invest. I do not have time to read them all, much less think about investing. Doctors do not receive any business training in medical school. We learn it on the fly in real world situations. It often feels overwhelming to find all these people coming at us to get us to buy their product or invest in their innovation.

There are marketers offering advice on how to sell and market to doctors specifically. The author of this post states that he laughs with someone who is faced with the task of marketing to doctors and feels their pain. He then goes on to give advice on how to get through to doctors. Apparently doctors refuse to use technology, such as voicemail and emails. (No, I just refuse to respond to things that don't interest me.) He reports that doctors have the most aggressive receptionists on the planet. (No offense but when I am treating patients I don't care about your product, no matter how awesome it may be.) The rest of his post is actually quite reasonable with the exception of the fact that he is trying to teach people to sell me things I don't want or need.[1]

Searching this topic, I found myriad advice on how to market to doctors, including YouTube videos. It rather amazes me that so much brainpower is devoted to this undertaking. Is it that they think doctors are rich and clueless? The actuality is that many people try to sell us stuff unsolicited. They drop in the office and ask for two minutes of my time. Trust me, if I can find an extra two minutes, I'm headed for the bathroom or brewing a cup of java. If I say I don't have time, I really mean that I don't have time. Don't keep arguing with me for two minutes because at that point, there really is NO way you will win a sale off me. I have had the marketer call the office calling pretending to be my personal bank reporting some kind of disaster. So if my staff gets me out of the exam room with a patient to answer your phone call trying to sell me something, well, all I can say is that you better wipe my phone number out of all your phone's memory banks and never call me again.

I do make appointments with sales reps and that is when I will listen to what you have to say. But it doesn't mean I am going to buy your product. Don't go thinking you own my soul because you brought me a tuna sandwich and Diet Coke. That is on you. I really don't care if I eat or not. If I say I am not interested, please don't keep calling me back. You will not change my mind. I will not have a sudden epiphany that I just have to buy your product. It is just annoying and I will probably start making fun of you with my office staff. I know you really want my business. But I am not just buying something to develop a business relationship with someone. It doesn't work that way.

It recently developed that people are looking to purchase doctors' practices again. Sure, you can make an offer. I witnessed very lucrative offers, which happen to be very unsustainable given the overhead expenses of the practice. Don't insult me by thinking I know nothing about business or that you know more about the business of running a

The War on Doctors

primary practice than I. You may have analyzed it and studied with a whole group of executives and consultants. You may have hired the biggest and the best. You may have earned a MBA with honors from an Ivy League college. But I live and breathe it every day. My livelihood depends on my knowledge of it. If it isn't working, I would not be able to survive. I know you want a piece of those profits. But please don't insult me by making an offer you cannot afford and pretending you know better than me. I can see right through you and you have just lost all my respect.

Then there are all the labs that come trying to get us to send all our blood (specimens, that is) to them. They offer to pay one of our staff as a phlebotomist. Well, that is against the Stark regulations. No, never. Giving you my business is not worth me losing my license over. This is not allowed by federal law. You expect me to break a federal law, punishable by fine and jail time, so you can earn my business? I must say this is a very bad way of trying to win me over to do business with you. I now think you are a criminal and am trying to distance myself from you as much as possible.

I never answer my home phone. More often than not, it is a recruiter trying to land me a lucrative job in some far-off location like Alaska. I am not searching for a new job, nor have I been looking for more than 10 years. Yet these calls continue unabated, despite multiple requests to be place on the Do-Not-Call list. The finder's fee for filling a position is quite lucrative. This makes many recruiters rather aggressive and persistent. No, I am not looking and am quite happy where I am. Many doctors no longer use recruiters to find employment just because of the hassle factor. They all want a piece of us to fill their wallets.

The representative from the Visiting Nurses' Association (VNA) stopped in the office for a friendly visit. She mentioned the fact that the VNA is currently purchasing doctors' practices. A few months ago, a hospital approached us to offer to buy our practice. This Wednesday, the family practice department meeting will discuss effective ways to sell a practice. Everyone wants to buy us out, it seems. It is not because they desire to get into the business of primary care and improve patients' lives. It is because they think they can make money from our work. Anyway, our practice is not for sale. Perhaps, when we get closer to retirement I would reconsider. But for now, I still have a long way to go and I turn down all the offers of those who not only want a piece of my practice, but actually want to take over the whole thing.

The banks want a piece of us, as well. They must perceive us as good debtors. We receive so many offers for business loans in our practice mailbox. Truth be told, they pretty much all head straight to the paper shredder. Some bankers just drop in the office or schedule a meeting to talk about their services. We have been offered all kinds of things, from lines of credit to credit card machines to refinancing the building that we practice in (which we are actually leasing and don't own). They all want a piece of our money.

Many companies need a doctor to be their director. There are many medical directors out there. Some of them do not even require the doctor to be physically on-site at the location they are medically directing. They just need that rank on their roles and a person with "MD" after their name to be able to sign papers that require a physician's signature. This role has been offered to me but I continually decline. I will not be the director of something that I am not actually directing.

All these situations consume our time. Doctors do not have enough time as it is. This attempt to kidnap our time for your own gain is a war on our time. We know you want to sell us something. That is your job. But it needs to be done in a respectful manner. This does not always happen. I once almost had to call the police to remove a salesperson from my office. He called me the next day to see if I was interested in his product. If I am not interested in buying your product, it is nothing against you personally. I just do not want your product, simple as that. It doesn't mean your product is bad, either. I just don't want it. We need to make these sales relationships more productive and stop wasting so much time. I am sure the salespeople would rather spend their time on people who are interested in purchasing their products. But do we really want to keep coming up with strategies to sell to uninterested doctors?

The War on Doctors

1-http://www.healthcaresuccess.com/marketing-to-doctors

Chapter 11 The Suits

Administrators are everywhere these days. Medicine has grown very top-heavy with executives. Executives in the insurance companies, hospitals, government agencies, JACHO, etc. Executives to make sure you discharge your patients when you are supposed to, executives to make sure you wash your hands the right way, executives to make sure you have a pleasant disposition in keeping compliant with JACHO guidelines. Oh, and let's not forget the executives at PQRS, HIPAA, MOC, CMS, and a whole alphabet of agencies. Pretty much if there is a job to be done, there are two or three suits to monitor the outcome and devise a strategic plan on how to improve it.

The following chart is quite revealing. If you examine it closely, you can see that the number of doctors in the US has increased very little since 1970. But just look at the explosion in healthcare administrators! After you're done with the glare of that eye-opening brightness, look at the line of expenditures in healthcare. It seems to mimic the rise in suits fairly closely. Looking at these numbers, it is obviously not the doctors driving the rising healthcare costs. In fact, it would be a good time to reiterate that perhaps we should downsize the number of bureaucrats in the system and the waste all this administration is costing and just let doctors practice medicine again.

The War on Doctors

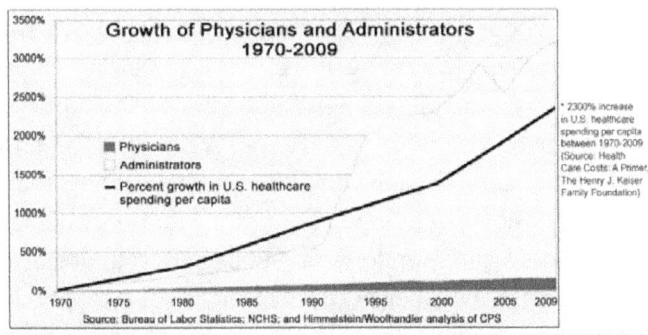

Growth of Physicians and Administrators
1970-2009

* 2300% increase in U.S. healthcare spending per capita between 1970-2009 (Source: Health Care Costs: A Primer, The Henry J. Kaiser Family Foundation)

Physicians
Administrators
— Percent growth in U.S. healthcare spending per capita

Source: Bureau of Labor Statistics; NCHS; and Himmelstein/Woolhandler analysis of CPS

"It is amazing that people who think we cannot afford to pay for doctors, hospitals, and medication, somehow think that we can afford to pay for doctors, hospitals, medication, and a government bureaucracy to administer it." –Thomas Sowell

1

These executives come with a high price tag attached. They earn far more than any doctor will ever hope to earn. Of course there are executives needed in the healthcare system. But there need to be limits. Most of these executives are not providing any direct patient care. They are not generating any revenue but are consuming it instead. They hold meetings and try to keep doctors up to certain benchmarks they determine from the guideline manual of the day. They determine protocols to push doctors to produce more, to ramp up their RVUs, to cut hospital costs. It requires many of them to make pretty charts to convince others it needs to be done and they try to develop laws to make sure it is done. Unfortunately, doctors just want to cure diseases and make people feel better. Sometimes, we cannot crank out 100s of RVUs from a patient encounter. Sometimes, we just need to lend our shoulder for the patient to cry on. There is no diagnostic code for that. The CPT codes fail us here. The administrators become irked when we see patients for things that do not generate revenue. This is causing a huge drain on the system, not just financially, but it is leading to doctors burning out. We cannot satisfy everyone. It is not humanly possible.

If we are forced to choose, we will pick our patients over the suits every time. This is why we spent years studying. This is why we answer our phones in the middle of the night. We sacrifice much for our patients' wellbeing. It is our calling. Dealing with administrators is not. It is more of a burden and hassle. We do not enjoy those meetings they force us to attend. We'd rather be in the office with our patients. Enough with this war of the useless requirements and supervision. Let us get back to caring for our patients and being doctors again. I am fortunate to be in private practice. I honestly do not know how many RVUs my work is equal to, nor do I care, and I expect I never shall. I am doing quite well administrating myself and I think doctors should be given more freedoms.

An article in the *NYT* speaks to the fact that doctors are not the top earners in the system, but rather finish in the middle of the pack. This article states that the top earners are those "overseeing the business of medicine." An analysis performed by the *NYT* by Compdata surveys revealed that the average salary of an insurance CEO was over $500,000 annually. The salary of a hospital CEO was over $300,000 per year, while that of a hospital administrator was around $237,000. In comparison, the average surgeon earned $306,000 while general medical doctors brought in approximately $185,000 annually. These numbers neglect the fact that the top earning executives often earn the bulk of their income in nonsalary compensation. For example, the CEO of Aetna, Mark Bertolini, earned a salary of $977,000 in 2012. However, his compensation package was well over $38 million in stocks vested and options he utilized that year. A hospital administrator of Barnabas Health, a medium-sized health system in NJ, earned a salary of $28,000 in 2012 but was compensated $21.7 million when he retired that same year. It is estimated that this proliferation of high earners in the healthcare system adds $2.7 trillion to the US healthcare bill every year. Other studies suggest that administrative costs comprise 20-30% of the healthcare spending in the US, far greater than in other countries.[2]

Is it fair to pick on the earnings of the top executives in medicine? Another article in *International Business Times* compared the salaries of these executives to those in other industries. Their analysis found that the salaries for these healthcare executives were higher than in any other industry in 2014. Those conducting this analysis showed that this is contributing to the rising healthcare costs. It was not just the executives in medicine that were found to earn an oversized paycheck, but managers just as well. This article points out a very important fact. There has been much debate about how to control the costs through such means as paying doctors only for quality rather than actual work and to cut out unnecessary ER visits. But there has never been any discussion on how to curb these exaggerated executive salaries. Another good point that was raised is that these executives are often additionally compensated in company stocks. This is a direct incentive to boost the value of those stocks by any means necessary. It was also estimated that US insurance companies pay twice as much on administrative costs than any other developed country.[3]

It is clear to see the conflict of interest the executives of these insurance companies possess. If they deny care or reduce services, the insurance company profits more, the stock value rises and they earn more money. Meanwhile, I stand in front of my patient and try to justify the fact that their MRI was denied although they probably tore their ACL. It is not about improving outcomes. It is not about helping patients get better or curing diseases. It is greed, plain and simple. Did you ever notice how the insurance companies develop their guidelines and formularies with little input from practicing physicians? It is because they know we would disagree with them. So while everyone is clamoring to reduce healthcare costs by changing to a pay-for-performance model, does anyone now believe that will really help? Go back and look at the chart. We need the executives to have oversight and stand up to their conflict of interest. We should not stand by while they suck the dollars out of the healthcare system directly into their own pockets. They need oversight. Someone needs to justify their earnings, because the statistics clearly do not. The healthcare workers encountering them do not. Isn't it time to go lean with the administration and put those dollars back into innovating medicine and curing diseases? Do we really want to watch them rake in the money while patients continue to suffer to try to get the care they need and deserve?

1- *Health Care Costs, A Primer*, The Henry J. Kaiser Family Foundation.
2- http://www.nytimes.com/2014/05/18/sunday-review/doctors-salaries-are-not-the-big-cost.html?_r=0
3- http://www.ibtimes.com/rising-costs-medical-care-health-insurance-median-pay-ceos-health-care-companies-1938699

Chapter 12 Physician Burnout

Wars cause casualties. The war on doctors is no different. Burnout rates are soaring and many physicians are leaving the practice of medicine. Worse yet, records show that approximately 300 doctors commit suicide every year.

There are new medical discoveries being made virtually every day. In addition to staying educated on these new findings, there are unique governmental regulations being rolled out all too frequently. These include meaningful use, NCQA, certified medical homes and others, which are all very time consuming and labor intensive. At the same time, insurance companies have required increasing amounts of paperwork and bureaucracy.

What is contributing to physician burnout?

- As stated above, rapidly advancing technologies and discoveries in medicine that we are expected to be aware of.
- Increased regulatory burdens from the government and insurance companies.
- Decreasing or stagnating incomes that do not adjust for rising overhead expenses or cost of living increases.
- Increased liability issues. This problem continues to flourish, allowing unneeded stress to be the backbone of much of what we do. Without tort reform and eliminating frivolous lawsuits, it will continue unchecked. Doctors pay high malpractice insurance premiums and many times feel much of medicine is done for defensive reasons.
- Increased denial of care is also a cause of our burnout. Increasingly, insurance companies are denying tests that doctors consider medically necessary. Prescribed medications are often not covered by a patient's prescription coverage. This is leading to an increasing feeling of helplessness among doctors. We are

trying to offer our patients the best medical care possible, yet often we feel our hands are tied by the insurance companies.

- Patients are increasingly unhappy. They are forced to buy their own premiums and facing higher deductibles, which they have to pay out-of-pocket. Frustration creeps in when they are unable to get the tests done that their doctor prescribed or take medications that they need.
- Life/work balance has been unbalanced. Doctors are working more hours than ever before. We are expected to take calls at night, on weekends and holidays. These are services that we often do not get paid to do. Yet many patients have no appreciation of this. It has become an expectation.
- Lack of solidarity among physicians. We often feel isolated and alone in our struggles. We do not see that other doctors are facing the same struggles that we are. This leads to isolation.

We are facing increasing changes in the healthcare field. Many physicians feel that we are expected to give more and more while we are getting less and less. This overwhelms many doctors, leading to burnout. Many of these factors are completely out of our control. We feel trapped in a system that we feel is not working and is in fact broken. We have little voice to speak up against many of the injustices we are seeing in this system. These feelings lead to burnout. More doctors are looking for alternative careers or to retire early. Many physicians are finding little enjoyment in their chosen profession. We need to get back to the system where doctors have a voice about what happens in medicine, a system where patients get the care they deserve.

In a recent *Medscape* article, it is noted that physicians are facing burnout like never before. In fact, we burn out more than any other profession in the US. In 2015 in the Medscape Physician Lifestyle Report, 46% of physicians responded that they suffered burnout. What do they define as burnout?

Burnout is commonly defined as loss of enthusiasm for work, feelings of cynicism, and a low sense of personal accomplishment. There have been questions about the use of these criteria, however. Some studies have suggested that a low sense of personal accomplishment is not associated with burnout, at least in men. In other research, simply including the statements "I feel burned out from my work" and "I have become more callous toward people since I took this job" appears to be a valid method for measuring burnout. Given the uncertainty in defining and measuring burnout, the criteria used in the Medscape survey to assess burnout in our physician members provide useful information on the current state of physician morale, which, unfortunately, is low. Furthermore, it was shown that those on the frontlines of medicine, ER doctors and primary care physicians, had the highest rates of burnout. Critical care physicians also had a high burnout rate. Interestingly the burnout rate among primary care doctors is not limited to the US only but is shown to be true in Europe as well.[1]

There are many serious consequences of physician burnout. One of the most important is substance abuse. According to this article, an average of 8-12% of doctors will face substance abuse at some point in their careers. This tends to mimic the rates in the general public. Even scarier are the statistics regarding physician suicide. Male doctors tend to commit suicide at twice the rate as men in the general public. Female physicians were three times as likely to commit suicide than other American women. Burnout also damages personal relationships.[2]

An article in the *NYT* discusses the widespread problem of physician burnout. Here it is mentioned that even medical students and doctors-in-training suffer burnout. It is estimated that approximately half of these young doctors face burnout at some point in their training. However, they are still under supervision so the consequences of their burnout are less likely to be as devastating. Researchers analyzed questionnaires from 7,000 doctors and found that "almost half complained about being emotionally exhausted, feeling detached from their patients, and work or suffering from a low sense of accomplishment." The researchers then compared this to 3,500 people working in other fields and adjusted it for age, sex, educational level and number of hours worked. They found the burnout rate among doctors significantly higher. Evaluating these numbers did not show any relationship to the number of hours worked or life-work balance. The only significant contributing factor appeared to be a specialty on the frontline of access to care, such as ER doctors and primary care specialists. According to the author of this article, this study points a grim picture of practicing medicine in the US. She suggests that the underlying mechanism for this burnout is doctors feeling trapped, with too little time to spend with patients and too many changing rules.[3]

In yet another survey of over 20,000 physicians, close to 50% reported being burned out. This article lists risks for burnout among physicians: "focusing on one's professional responsibilities obsessively, excessive workload, lack of sleep, and 'frontline' exposure to patients such as experienced in primary care and emergency departments. Difficult interactions with patients with unrealistic expectations, demands of healthcare system administrators for productivity, added government regulatory requirements including use of an electronic health record, anguish over medical liability cases, and new requirements for maintenance of board certification could also be contributory factors." The extreme consequences of burnout lead to depression and even suicide. Another suggested factor is that doctors are no longer the respected professionals that they used to be. One reason that doctors are more likely to successfully commit suicide than those in other professions is the fact that they have ready access to the lethal means of doing so.[4]

Another article proposes that physician burnout is the inevitable consequence of maladaptive behaviors learned in medical education. In medical school, technical skills needed for the student to become a doctor are taught with little attention given to learning interpersonal skills. This fails to prepare students for the reality of practicing medicine. The hidden agenda in medical school values performance and competition over collaboration. Additionally, little training is given on how to be a leader or an effective member of an organization. Another factor contributing to burnout among doctors is the value of presenteeism. Doctors are driven to be present at work no matter what, no matter how sick.[5]

There are many studies and articles examining the issue of physician burnout. They all tend to find it more common in the frontline specialties and most propose the same causative factors. Loss of autonomy is a big one. Much of what we do as doctors these days is being wrenched from our hands and being decided by third parties from insurance companies and governmental employees. Many of these decisions are senseless and not in the best interests of patients. We know that they are decisions derived to reduce healthcare costs and increase profits to insurance companies. But our pleas to help our patients increasingly fall on deaf ears. In my area, there is a big shortage of primary doctors and I struggle to accept as many new patients as is physically possible. While the crush of work grows, the mandates taking us away from this work increase as well. It is a wonder that not all doctors are burning out.

There is also a plethora of seminars, articles and other sources on how to treat physician burnout. Of course, all these are promoting their own products and cost money. Can spending a wad of money on a feel-good video help? Or is it just another entity trying to feed off our distress? There are many suggestions and tips to heal our burnout, telling us how to heal ourselves. But is this even possible when the problems inherent in our system still persist unabated? Sure, spending a week in a happy conference would feel good; it is a week off work, after all. But then we go back to the same situations that caused us to burnout in the first place.

So how do we correct burnout, then? In my mind, the only real lasting way is to change the system. While I know this is an enormous undertaking, it is the only way to give us back our autonomy and freedom to practice medicine in the way we feel is the best for our patients. We need to be more connected with each other if we want to make any effective changes. In an isolated state, we have failed. We need to fight the injustices in the system. As long as we are forced to continue swallowing the bitter pill, our insides will burn. We need to speak up and speak out any chance that we find. Doctors deserve their respect back. Patients deserve their humanity back. No less is acceptable. Even if I rage into the night alone, I will continue this fight against the war of injustice inflicted on doctors and patients alike. Into the bitter winter of medicine, I raise my voice.

1- http://www.medscape.com/viewarticle/838437
2- http://www.eric.vcu.edu/home/resources/pipc/Other/Clinical_Ski lls/Article_Physician_Burnout.pdf
3- http://well.blogs.nytimes.com/2012/08/23/the-widespread-problem-of-doctor-burnout/?_r=0
4- http://www.philly.com/philly/blogs/fieldclinic/Physician-burnout-and-suicide-the-postmodern-doctors-dilemma.html
5- http://www.sciencedirect.com/science/article/pii/S22130586140 00084

The War on Doctors

Conclusion

Medicine as we know it will soon end. Too many hands are trying to control the wheel of our healthcare destination. This will only lead us to a big crash and we will need to reinvent ourselves or be taken over as tools of the trade. Doctors are leaving medicine and the ones staying are losing hope. How long can we wage this war and try to win the best for our patients?

Over the past several years, the war on doctors evolved. Healthcare spending in the US represents the biggest expenditure in our economy, and everyone wants a piece of the money pot. Doctors leave the profession in larger numbers as the projected shortage intensifies. The power to practice medicine is being wrenched from doctors' hands by third parties in many sectors. But the war on doctors to gain control of the industry is not devastating doctors alone. The war on doctors is a war on patients as well. Unless this battle is ended, both physicians and patients will suffer.

Who is at war with doctors?

Third party insurance companies cause the biggest devastation in the practice of medicine. They do not put patients first but rather are driven by lust for their own profits. The average annual salary of an insurance company CEO is over 10 million dollars. Yet patients struggle to get the insurance companies to cover even the costs of many of their generic medications. There are certain diagnostic tests that will not even be considered without special permission from an insurance company employee. So despite doctors ordering tests they know will benefit their patients' health or even save their lives, these tests will only be performed with the blessing of an insurance company clerk. Doctors are losing this battle. I see this in my practice every day and it just keeps getting worse and worse. How do you comfort a patient who is crying because their insurance company refuses to cover their MRI and they believe they suffer from brain cancer? And as their doctor, you examined them and saw signs that made you suspicious that they may be right. The doctors bear the full brunt of liability in the case of missed diagnoses, even when we try to do right by the patient. Insurance companies and their employees are exempt from any liability for their decisions. They claim they do not practice medicine. I disagree. When they usurp my medical decisions that I made after carefully examining my patients and taking their histories, and calculate that all through the filter of my education and training, they have made a decision and it affects the health of my patients.

The government is another big warrior in this war on doctors. Many of the frustrations patients feel in the exam rooms are the direct result of new laws and mandates flowing out of the halls of Congress. Do you know how patients hate that doctors spend the office visit looking at their computer screens? Well, doctors hate it even more. The HITECH act, signed into law in 2009, set in motion the widespread use of EHRs. While tech is good and the need for legible and transferable records clear, this act also set into play many other mandates. The meaningful use program quickly followed, which was heralded to be a means to test that doctors use their EHR in a meaningful. Unfortunately, that meaningful way was determined by the government, not the users of the EHR systems. So of course, these mandates ended up being onerous and useless. While a patient is upset that the doctor is not looking at them, the doctor is more annoyed that they must input numerous unnecessary information into the medical record. And if we don't? This year it went into effect that any doctor not participating in the meaningful use program will be penalized a percentage of their Medicare reimbursements. These penalties will increase every year. We own no opinion in this. We protested and explained how this is interfering in our practice of medicine. The governmental ears remain stone deaf.

There is also a **media** war on doctors. When you think of all the times you hear doctors mentioned in the news, what comes to mind? There are stories of wrongful surgeries, medication errors, greedy doctors and those who lost their license to practice medicine. How often do you hear tales of the good doctors do? Doctors are saving lives as we speak. They are missing their kid's ballet recitals and family reunions to do this. While most people sleep through the night, doctors have their mobiles on the ready on their dressers and night stands to answer calls at any time. There is nothing called 9-5 in medicine. I go home when I am finished taking care of my patients. I may get phone calls for the rest of the night when I go home. Most doctors still treat Medicaid patients, for which we get paid very little. In fact, we are lucky to break even financially on these patients. Yet we do it out of a sense of calling because we believe being a doctor is a noble profession and it is a calling more than a job. Do you know that doctors lose sleep and cry over our patients? It is a very frequent occurrence but we do it behind the scenes because it is necessary to appear strong in front of our patients. They need our strength even when we don't have any left. But the media stereotype doesn't allow patients to see this side of us.

How is the war on doctors a war on patients?

When a patient can't get a test or medication they need because the insurance company refuses to cover it, they can be harmed. A patient and her doctors fought the insurance company to cover a brain MRI because she was having suspicious neurological symptoms. She was told that it was not a medical decision, just a determination of benefits, and that she could pay out-of-pocket. This woman is a single mother putting two kids through college and working 12 hours a day. She did not have the money and she simply could not do any more to get the amount that was needed. After almost 12 months of appeals she finally got the MRI approved. Sadly, her brain tumor was finally diagnosed. This is only one patient but every doctor has scores of these stories. Real harm can happen and will happen unless doctors are again allowed to make the medical decisions they need for their patients. Insurance companies and their employees need to start bearing some responsibility and liability for the decisions they are making, without examining patients or even talking to them. Doctors cannot keep practicing like this and patients deserve better, especially when many of them are now paying their own insurance premiums.

The mandates doctors are forced to comply with are taking time away from patients. In the 21st century, patients are living longer and suffering from more complex diseases. They need our time more than ever. When we cannot give them the time they need because we are busy playing data entry clerk for Uncle Sam, their care will be sub-optimal. It is time to get the politicians out of the exam room and let the doctors and patients be a team again. The governmental intrusion into the health of its citizens will have far-reaching and adverse consequences. We need to win this fight before more casualties result.

When people heed media stereotypes of doctors, a fissure develops in the doctor-patient trust. We need to trust each other in order to achieve the best clinical outcomes. Doctors need to trust that patients give us accurate information. Patients need to trust that we hold their best interests at heart. The media casts doctors in a negative light and people see us as driven for profit. A patient asked me for a medication that I believed would harm her because of her medical problems. She became upset and accused me of not wanting to help her because I get paid less under Obamacare. Truthfully, I personally (I am not sure if this is true across the board for primary care doctors) actually get paid the same from most plans and slightly more under Medicare and Medicaid. But the assumption was there. Sure, there are outliers. But most doctors love our patients. We need more balanced stories about good things that doctors do and not just the bad apples.

The war on doctors is happening on many fronts. Doctors are getting burned out trying to give our patients the best medical care while fighting all these wars. Those waging the battle against us possess all the power in this war. They own the healthcare dollar and where it will go. They hold power over us in the ability to perform our chosen careers. We are losing this war because we cannot fight back individually. Doctors need to join together and speak out about the evils in the system. Patients need to join us before these powers lead to very real harms. It may seem like a gargantuan task. But remember, David beat Goliath in the end. It is time that good returns to medicine.

www.ingramcontent.com/pod-product-compliance
Lightning Source LLC
Chambersburg PA
CBHW070908180526
45168CB00005B/1973